My Body Is a Big Fat Temple

AN ORDINARY STORY OF PREGNANCY AND EARLY MOTHERHOOD

Alena Dillon

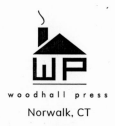

woodhall press

Norwalk, CT

Versions of select chapters originally appeared in the following publications: Scary Mommy, The VIDA Review, The Smart Set, and Mothers Always Write.

Library of Congress Cataloguing-in-Publication Data available

ISBN

First Edition

Woodhall Press, 81 Old Saugatuck Road, Norwalk, CT 06855
WoodhallPress.com
Distributed by IPG"

Dear Rowen,

I was a hapless gardener who scattered seeds without expectation, only to one morning discover a proliferation of daylilies, azalea, lavender, peonies, dahlia, honeysuckle, and marigold. You are my bounty of joy. You dazzle me.

Mimi

PREFACE

Dear Readers,

My mother is a map person—hard copy, because digital will not do. She drives with spiral-bound, laminated books charting the tristate area in the compartment of her car door. She stood below the Arc de Triomphe and ironed creases from one she tore from a travel guide. She's the first person in a decade to walk into the City Hall of Beverly, Massachusetts, where I live, to request a paper map, compelling the municipal employee to sift through a filing cabinet until he found a document from a simpler time, yellowed with age. I imagine him blowing dust from its surface like a cinematic scholar who stumbled upon an antique book he didn't realize was cursed, though the audience sure did.

Navigation is not my strength. When a group gathers around a phone to consider their route on Google Maps, I'm the one murmuring my consideration while also drifting farther back. But I can relate to the impulse to orient oneself, to clarify one's my sense of direction. My maps, though, are books, and the experiences they share. Through them, I find my way. Without them, the world drops out of sight and, unsure how to proceed, or even how to feel, I freeze.

When embarking on unfamiliar terrain, I am as insistent as my mother. But instead of waving away my brother's iPhone as we traverse the winding streets of the North End—she doesn't need his app because she has a map—I scour libraries and bookstores. Those who have come before warn what to expect, and how many granola bars to pack. (The whole box. Always the whole box.) But more than that, I collect company so I don't have to travel alone.

I hunted for comrades inside bindings the moment my husband and I considered starting a family. There were pregnancy guides and how-to parenting books, as well as investigations of prenatal topics I referenced as bibles (Expecting Better,

Like a Mother) *but not as many exploring the personal experience. There were a few*—Great with Child, Waiting for Birdy, Operating Instructions, Homing Instincts, Maybe Baby, *among others. I nested with these authors the way other women are said to alphabetize spice racks and sanitize ice cube trays to prepare their households. I was preparing my mind, cultivating gumption and know-how. Pregnancy is so variable, I wanted an army of women to swap perspectives, trials, fears, and joys to increase the odds of discovering myself in the pages. But despite being imperative to our species, pregnancy is not given much shelf space.*

Nonfiction is a tricky genre, often requiring a strong platform, or at least a catchy hook. In other words, the author must be famous or have undergone an astonishing experience. There is certainly a place for celebrity memoir and harrowing tales. I've been known to double fist them. But standard experiences reflect the struggles and delights typical to the average Jo-sephine. They mirror the human heart. There is relief in discovering a shared humanity and realizing you are not alone. Or, as the poet Adrienne Rich phrased it in her book Of Woman Born, *"the willingness to share private and sometimes painful experience can enable women to create a collective description of the world which will truly be ours." Besides, even the most typical accounts of pregnancy and motherhood are extraordinary, and extraordinarily harrowing (spoiler alert).*

The general public might not realize this because conversations about pregnancy are often airbrushed. We crop out the ugly parts, smudge over the distasteful, and enhance the romantic. In the rare instances when we speak honestly, it is in hushed tones so no one hears the secret: it kinda sucks. Why the discretion? Because lady-bit chitchat is impolite, or at least uninteresting, especially to those without that brand of bit. Also, we wouldn't want the truth to intimidate women with still vacant wombs.

I was reminded of this when, legs parted on an exam table, I wailed, "Why didn't anybody warn me?" and a medical practitioner answered, "If you knew, you never would have gotten pregnant." She's lucky I didn't harness my pregnancy hormones and barrel gut to bulldoze her into a flap of white coat and regret.

Women don't need to be tricked. Despite being silenced, harassed, and repressed; despite having to bear and raise children; despite being responsible for household duties; despite being invited into the workforce during World War II, offered universal childcare, and having all that ripped away; despite unpaid maternity leave, wage disparities, and corporate locker-room talk; despite being called hysterical or frigid, unreasonable or bossy, overly emotional or bitchy; despite having to coddle the male ego; despite cramps, Spanx, and underwire; despite all that's worked against us—we run the world, or at least Beyoncé does. We deserve respect, knowledge, and transparency. Imagine if doctors didn't divulge the reality of a vasectomy to a male patient, and when, cradling sore testicles, he demanded to know why he wasn't informed beforehand, the doctor answered brightly, "If I'd told you, you never would have had the procedure!"

Besides, there are women with more than one child—lots of them. We live through pregnancy and for some reason agree to get pregnant again.

This is the type of book I was looking for, more than prenatal vitamins and ovulation trackers, and I figure there are other women out there who are hungry for information, honesty, and community the way yogurt commercials depict us as being hungry for 100-calorie dessert substitutes. I hope I can contribute to somebody's network with this collection, and that one day I too will find an orgasm in the dairy section.

Each of these essays was written from inside the experience or, if that was impractical, directly following it. I wasn't jotting notes in the midst of contractions, for example. I sought to capture my emotions like lightning bugs in glass jars before their charge faded, or was buffed or dulled by retrospect. I wrote while fearful, excited, awed, grieved, pissed off, and desperately needing to pee. I wrote while I was childless, expecting, as a new mother, and then as a slightly less new one. The voice of the narrator evolves along the way because, over this three-year maternal passage, including as our world was struck by plague, I evolved. (Sometimes, when appropriate, a future me returned to the text to intersperse moments of foreshadowing.)

Even as a female—a feminist female—it took being pregnant for me to revere women's true resilience and mystical capabilities. I never appreciated how incredibly demanding the feat of creation is, the toll it takes on the body and mind, and how arduous it is to continue through the motions of life while forming one inside you. If I saw a pregnant woman on the subway, I didn't comprehend she might have diabetes for the first time in her life. When I sat beside her in the waiting area of our OB-GYN, I didn't consider the fortitude required when dreading bad news. When I noticed her in a diner booth, I didn't acknowledge that bacon grease was an olfactory finger down her throat, yet she braved breakfast with her family anyway. I never appreciated her grit and valor. Her divine strength. Her supernatural gift. I saw her without seeing her.

Girl, I see you now, and not just because you are growing larger by the day. Because you are larger than life. You are, in fact, two lives.

This is for the pregnant, the famished, and the tired. It's for you who have nibbled the same brand of cracker for the last three weeks because it's just the right crispness and anything more or less will make you heave. It's for you who want to call out of work but can't afford to take another sick day, though you've never been so sick in your life. It's for you with pain shooting into your crotch and tightness in back and belly muscles you didn't know you had. It's for you whose swollen ankles have amalgamated with your calves, and whose shoes may never fit again. It's for you who have grown a two-pound organ, just for this occasion, that will be the second rider out the log chute. It's for you who can't soothe your newborn from the kind of open-mouthed howling that is so furious, so despaired, he stops breathing for a second, and so do you. It's for you who are so overwhelmed by maternity you can't remember who else you are. It's for you who expected motherhood to be different, and worry it will never get better. It's for you who want to be a mother—even if only sometimes—and for you who don't.

I wrote this to process why I was afraid, stressed, frustrated, uncomfortable, hopeful, fractured, and amazed by pregnancy and preliminary parenthood, and why those feelings mattered to me and to our collective human experience. Call it therapy, academic inquiry, my craft, my living. Call it whatever you want—here it is, and I hope it honors the struggle that is necessary to the survival of our kind, but that is so often overlooked, underappreciated, shrugged off, or forgotten completely.

Sincerely,

Writer, Wife, Daughter, Sister, Friend, Mother, Me

PART I

Pre-Pregnancy

Puppy Love

PEOPLE SAY DOGS ARE THE GATEWAY DRUGS TO HAVING A BABY, BUT THAT'S not why we adopt our little doobie. We adopt her because I'm tired of strolling around town, realizing my husband isn't beside me anymore, and spinning around to find he's kneeling on the sidewalk two blocks back, nose to nose with a golden retriever. That guy is constantly chasing tail.

Penelope Chews—Penny for short—is lanky and floppy, with big paws, ears, and a tongue she'll never grow into, a fourteen-pound labhound mix rescued with her siblings from a cardboard box on the Kentucky roadside. When Phil cradles her against his chest, she licks his chin like she already knows she's his. Soon we'll learn she's saying, "Sorry, pal, I have a belly full of parasites, so prepare for my ass to explode over your backyard for the next three months."

There are joys of dog ownership: When she learns a trick, or half a trick, since we have to modify our sweet dummy's "roll over" to "dead fish." When her tail pendulums in greeting. When we take her for a run, and she grabs the leash in her mouth to slow Phil down because I'm huffing twenty feet behind, patting my pockets for my inhaler. When her velvet ears shift back on her head like a sail adjusting to the wind, or perk up into silky quotation marks, framing thoughts of *BONE! TREAT! SQUIRREL!* When the light yellows her eyes into sleepy wolf slits. When she circles next to me and drops into a tired pile against my thigh. When she trots to her dog dish at five o'clock sharp. She tells time better than most millennials.

But at the risk of sounding like a garbage-person, there are also days when I don't particularly like Penny.

On Thanksgiving, Penny frolics on my parents' property, or what we call Penny's country house, alongside my older brother's infinitely energetic border collie and my parent's more crotchety cockapoo. There are not many more idyllic sights than dogs unleashed.

We lose sight of her around a bush, and that is all it takes for her to surface the knob of an ancient ham bone my parents' dog buried an unknown number of weeks, months, or years ago. She parades it before us, her head held high, trotting like a dressage horse. The bone fragment is the size of a tennis ball, gray, and clotted with dirt. It's hard to tell what phase of decomposition has been interrupted, but I'd wager somewhere between mob-hit-washed-ashore and fossil.

Phil fishes a handful of kibble from his pocket and extends his hand. "Penny, come." He sounds breezy, like he isn't after her treasure; he wants to give her *more* food. He's disturbingly convincing—the Russian spy of dog training.

Penny cocks her head. She's not entirely persuaded, but that kibble sure does look tempting, sitting right there in Phil's palm, free of charge. It'd be rude to turn down such a generous offer. She steps forward, her stare locked on the treats. Then she eyes Phil once more. Finally, she drops the ham bone, pounces on the dog food, and laps it up. I sigh. Crisis averted. Then she dives back to the bone. Before Phil has the chance to react, she grabs the decaying matter in her maw, unhinges her jaw, and swallows it whole.

Our six-month-old puppy-python returns to her sniffing, completely unaware that a fist of cartilage is barreling through her system. We stare, speechless, petrified it will, at any moment, rip her esophagus, lodge in her stomach, or obstruct her bowel. There's nothing we can do but wait. I can't engage with the rest of the family gathering. I'm too busy assessing Penny's behavior. Is she lying on the couch because she's tired from play, or is her lethargy a symptom? Are her eyes droopy? Yes, they are definitely droopy. Should we tear a veterinarian from her holiday just to have her tell us that Penny is presenting with hound eyes because she's a hound?

At the sound of her retching, Phil and I fly out of bed, fight the crate open, and carry Penny outside in time for her next bout. There, in the stillness of two in the morning, we watch her be sick for five hours.

Penny, the heaving soloist, is accompanied by a symphony of rustling leaves, hooting owls, and screeching fisher-cats. There's something contemplative about the dead of the night, when you're standing in the dark, the sky pricked by stars and illuminated by a crescent moon, knowing most people within hundreds of miles are asleep, while your dog pukes in the dewy grass at your feet. It makes you wonder, *Remember when holidays were easier? What are we doing? And dear Lord was that hot mud or dog barf?* (It's never hot mud. There *is* no hot mud.)

The next day, while we play UNO with our own customized family rules, including holding our breath and discarding Reverses from behind our backs, I'm too exhausted and preoccupied to even contribute to Mega Draw Four. What does the persisting vomit and diarrhea mean? Has Penny digested the bone yet? Will she be okay?

Was getting a dog a mistake?

• • • • •

Penny looms over us at six in the morning, her tiger-eye irises a set of black marbles in the dark, peering down at her drooling, snoring, slumberous owners like, "So, uh, you guys are awake, right?"

Phil stirs into consciousness, squints, and scratches her ear. "Morning, you little scamp." Then he follows her into the living room where he spots a pile of gray cloth he mistakes for the mangle of his Irish flatcap. "Oh man."

Phil doesn't value many material goods. He'd be amenable to donating everything save for his electric guitar, wedding ring, utility knife, two pairs of boxers, and his Irish flatcap. Ireland is the landscape equivalent of his personality with its rolling, unpopulated countryside, gray skies, and misty glens. He cherishes that cap, and wears it everywhere but the shower. It would be a big deal if Penny destroyed it.

I sit up in bed, sensing my husband might finally lose his patience. Shit is about to go down.

But his tone lilts back up. "False alarm. It's a wool sock. But even if it was my hat, I'd already forgiven her."

He thought she had chewed up his favorite thing, and he'd forgiven her instantly.

Phil's temperament should bolster my confidence in our ability to parent—after all, he'll be half of my team. He has his flaws, like anybody else—he can go through an entire day forgetting to brush his teeth, his sense of style can be best described as "wool," and he considers the original *MacGyver* to be good television—but his patience makes it easy to imagine him flourishing as a father. Our children might draw on the walls, scream in the car, mash Goldfish with balled-up fists, or cross their arms over their chest, and Phil will react with tolerance and strategy. He'll extend the metaphorical kibble. He might pull a plaid shirt over their striped pants, torture them with cheesy shows about a resourceful haircut, or approach their heartache with the emotional deftness (oops, I meant deafness) he's applied to my own breakdowns, saying, "I can see you're upset," when steam is straight-up whistling out of my ears, but he'll also forgive them instantly.

What about me?

I tend to relationships like a horticulturist to her gardenia. (The following is strictly a metaphor for how I love *people*. I'm homicidal when it comes to actual plants. I've killed air plants, and they don't even need soil. A gardenia would take one look at me and hari-kari itself into the earth.) I spray daily, position planters at big windows and rotate them by the hour. I ask questions and log the answers. I worry over their responses and my own. I follow up. I set dates. I cultivate connections until buds open and expand to fill my brain space.

But having Penny has surfaced an unsettling realization about my attachment style: my capacity to love and to love hard comes with a built-in delay. I'm not sure I love our dog yet, or not always, or at least not always well enough.

I'm preparing for company when Penny makes eye contact, squats, and looses a fire hose of piss whose longevity is only possible if Jesus has diversified his never-ending fish trick to include puppy bladders.

As I retrieve rug cleaner for my little miracle worker, the rice boils over on the stove. I lift the pot off the burner while Penny canters through her urine and tracks it into the living room. I shoo her and blot the mess with paper towels. Then I smell something charring. The Brussels sprouts are under the broiler. I leap into the kitchen, and Penny scurries back, tears up the soiled towels, and scatters them around the apartment.

I grab her by the scruff and scold through gritted teeth. "No!"

I hear a flash of my mother from when I was a kid. *I used to be a nice person. A fun person.*

I finally understand what she meant, because I used to be a nice person, a fun person. Now look at me: I'm wrenching a puppy's collar.

· · · · ·

All in one week, Penny dives for a leaf while I tie her poop bag, and the contents upend like filthy confetti; she tears my new yoga pants; she eats our neighbor's dog poop, which gives her *another* round of parasites; I wrestle a detached squirrel tail from her jaws; a man offers a treat to his dog, and Penny charges him, her front paws propelling into his crotch as if his groin has a bull's-eye. (Okay, that one is kind of funny.)

I pet her only cordially, which saddens Phil. He asks, "Have you forgiven Penny yet? Do you love her again?"

"Not yet," I say, and I'm only partly kidding.

Then, while Penny is clipped into her lead behind our apartment, she accidentally wraps herself around the pole of a poop bag dispenser. She realizes that she is trapped and darts the wrong way around the pole, tying herself tighter. She braces her front paws against the dirt and yanks her neck back over and over, desperate to free herself, her eyes wide with terror, her hackles rising like crow feathers.

All at once, my Grinch heart grows three sizes. I throw open the sliding glass door and dash across the wet grass, calling, "It's okay, Penny. You're okay." When she sees me, it's as if she recognizes that I am a person who takes care of her, and she calms.

It's a wonder, no small miracle, that a creature of a different species, someone who doesn't look like me, act like me, or communicate like me, someone who was involuntarily thrust into my possession, could trust me so quickly and completely, could love me, miss me, rely on me, and consider herself part of my pack.

I unclip her from the lead, scoop her into my arms, and carry her inside, where I sit on the floor, where so many of her accidents have discolored the carpet, and pull her against me. She lets herself be guided and drops her weight, and I stroke the fur on her back. Only then do I realize my socks are muddy, ruined, and that my heart is pounding. I don't care about all the ways she's been naughty. Here we are in consecrated communion, intrinsically connected, dependent on one another for affection and protection, a woman and her dog. She is my girl and I am hers. I love her, and forgive her instantly.

* * * * *

Penny and I have been in sync for years, but I worry I love her better simply because, being older and more behaved, she's easier to love, and it isn't enough to love someone when she's being good. Children often aren't good, and that's fine; they shouldn't have to behave to earn your favor, just as you shouldn't love someone only because they show you love. And yet, when I open the bathroom door to find Penny on the other side, eyes rounded, waiting for me, my heart swells. "Good girl," I say. "Good girl."

＊ ＊ ＊ ＊ ＊

As I write this, I'm balanced on the edge of the couch with Penny sprawled behind me, her head resting on a pillow, lightly snoring. Her back legs are curled up against her belly and her front legs are pointed straight, mummyesque, as if feeling her way through the dark. When sunlight reflects off the crooks of her ears and cheekbones, it shimmers a dusky spectrum. But here, away from the window, her fur is immaculately black. Our velveteen panther.

At times like this, when her body is coiled around mine, she feels like my daemon, my spirit incarnated as a canine. I match my breath to hers and am happy to act as her warden while she sleeps, just as she often stands guard at our back door, muscles tensed, eyes alert, our panting sentry. If a bird or squirrel wants to get to us, it'll have to be through her. But here, on the couch, I take my turn as steward.

She often looks like a stuffed animal, so divine she must have been manufactured, like those black lab puppies children lift from red-ribboned boxes Christmas morning. Sometimes the sight of her inflates me. I don't mind that her hair finds its way everywhere: into my laptop keys, the bathtub, my coffee. Or that I have to handle turds on a daily basis with a too-thin layer of plastic separating them from my skin, which isn't enough to conceal their warmth. Or that I've become as committed to dog walking as the United States Postal Service is to mail delivery: neither snow nor rain nor heat nor gloom of night stays this walker from the swift completion of her appointed round.

I realize raising a dog is easier than raising children. When I lose my temper, yanking her away from the open dishwasher, when I leave her alone for more hours than I should, she forgets. Dogs are beautiful beasts, not just because of the grace with which they sprint, the leather of that finely cut nose, their padded paws, the human expressiveness of their eyebrows, or the downy place around their whiskers. They're beautiful because they don't hold grudges. They don't manipulate. They don't get sick of your annoying habits or tire of your love. They lay their whole selves at your feet. They are happy to see you.

They are grateful for that same cup of cheap dry food they've scarfed down the last thousand days. They don't know, or at least don't seem to resent, that of their two owners, you're the impatient one.

Children aren't so lenient. Mine will remember when I lost my temper, just as I remember when my mother lost hers. I will be held accountable.

But perhaps it is that trepidation, that risk, that makes human love sacrosanct. It must be earned. A dog will always love you, but humans can withdraw, screen phone calls, skip holidays, ignore, scorn, and move away. Or we can open ourselves up, be vulnerable, focus on the ways someone loves well rather than their shortcomings. We can cherish the good times and have mercy for the bad. We can come together and create a new life, and pray that person will grow up to forgive and love as you have forgiven and loved.

• • • • •

Penny often got sick as a puppy—leave it to us to adopt not just a dog, but all her parasite friends—but we've been fortunate on the destructive chewing front. The only item she ever destroyed was a paperback book, which she pulled from the coffee table and systematically shred to pieces. The book was Cesar Millan's *How to Raise the Perfect Dog*.

I like to think she gets her sense of irony from me.

What to Expect When You're Expected to Expect

MY GRANDFATHER IS A CLEAN-SHAVEN, DIABETIC SANTA CLAUS, A RETIRED leprechaun with eyes the stark blue of a sky following a blizzard and a suit in every color—I mean *every* color—that he wears on a rotating schedule, using a color wheel pocket square he folds to appear blue or green or yellow, and therefore wearable with all of his suits. He fills parking meters about to expire. He knows the name of every employee at the diner he frequents. He grabs my elbow before crossing the street, even though I'm a grown-ass woman.

I don't know how you get to be eighty-nine without the world stomping your goodness, but he's managed, though he's experienced his share of misfortune: an alcoholic father, his mother's leg amputation, the death of his wife of sixty years—a loss that devastated him. But even that pain produced grief so uncontaminated it's almost too tender to exist in this world. He talks to her every night, providing her a recap of the day's events. He holds her government-issued ID in his hand while he sleeps, and every morning he carries that ID to the window and says, "Good morning, Joan. This is what today looks like."

Because of his virtues, I don't fault him when he tells me, "I can't wait until you call me with good news. May Phil's men find their target tonight," or when he wrote in a card, "I am 'expecting' you'll have a great anniversary!" and underlined the word three times to guide his implication with the subtlety of an air traffic controller. It comes from a wholesome place, since he's wholesome all the way through—he just *assumes* I'm trying to have kids. This is the expectation of all married women of a certain age. I don't tell him it would be a miracle almost equal to the Immaculate Conception, since I've taken as much birth control as they'll legally prescribe.

I like my childless marriage. My husband and I work side by side at our kitchen table, cook together, and explore the North Shore of Boston: sandy coves, orchards, wood trails, breweries, seafood shacks, and fishing villages. In the summer, we adventure abroad: ferrying Scandinavian fjords, hiking the Canadian Rockies, meandering Ireland's country roads, or traveling to a new city, where each morning in Charleston, Paris, San Francisco, or Montreal, we stroll cobblestone streets, sip cappuccinos at a café, or wander a waterfront district. We drift untethered. We answer to no one. We explore at our whim, light and free, bound to no schedules, needs, or desires but our own (and those of our dog, whom we take where we can). Perhaps because of this pleasant existence, this general ease, we are kind to one another.

Relaxed relationships often seize up under the strain of children, as couples engage in a partner juggling act of swords, fire, and sleep schedules, attempting to socialize while shoveling food into their mouths and the mouths of all their dependents, wrangling tantrums, or debating in tense civility (because others are watching) whether that week they are enforcing the Positive Parenting or Unconditional Parenting strategy.

Bitterness becomes more natural to dish out with practice, and can corrode affection away until there's nothing left but hostility that's passed around the dinner table as easily as the mashed potatoes. Some couples become so accustomed to meanness they grow calluses. I don't want calluses. I want to be kind to my friend.

Phil and I compliment a well-made meal. We express thanks when the dishes are cleaned or the water bill is paid. We are silly, call each other Bub, speak in a language of our own invention, and create spoof lyrics to popular songs, like a Daylight Saving Time riff off Bruno Mars's "Uptown Funk." *Don't believe your wristwatch.* We walk our dog and hash out our days, listening with full attention and offering advice. Phil inspires me to be more easygoing and honest, and I force him to socialize when his instinct is to stay home and watch a fire burn on YouTube since we don't have a fireplace.

Childless couples report higher rates of happiness. If I'm going to risk my happy life and marriage, it should be for something we definitely want, and not just because my eggs are spoiling as we speak and I don't want a geriatric pregnancy, which—absurdly, unfairly, *rudely*—begins at thirty-five.

The hope is that becoming parents will intensify and add a rich complexity to our relationship. The fear is that it will take a big ol' baby poop on it.

In my nightmare, a tomato-faced baby screams in one arm while I warm a bottle of milk and Penny barks at the mailman and I snap at Phil, "Are you just going to sit there?"

I see us on barstools at the kitchen counter, crunching cereal in silence, remembering foggily how we used to dance to fiddle music while turkey bacon and cinnamon pancakes sizzled on a skillet. I see us asking, "How was your day?" without caring about the answer, or not asking it at all. I see our bodies pivoting in the hall so we pass one another without touching. These are chilling visions. I don't want to resent the husband I enjoy. I don't want to become angry and tired, bored and boring. We're happy. Is it wise to mess with happiness?

• • • • •

My dad loves babies enough to make strangers nervous. If he gets one in his arms, he sways. His mustache tickles their cheek until their eyelids droop, unperturbed by their new six-foot height, and they sleep.

His zeal does not threaten a mother on a flight to Arizona. As he walks down the aisle to the bathroom, he passes her with her infant and toddler. Because he's learned how it sounds when a man is interested in children, he says, "My wife would love to hold that baby." It's creepy as hell, but the mother replies, "Tell her to come down anytime." My father returns to his seat and tells my mother, who proceeds down the aisle. The woman says, "Are you the one who wants to hold my baby?" (So creepy.) And, "Do you want to take her to your seat?" (Seriously, who is this lady?) My mother carries the infant to the opposite end of the plane, and she and my father take turns holding it for the remaining two hours. When the pilot announces he is preparing for landing, my mother carries the infant to the back, where she finds the mother drooling against the windowpane. If you've ever wondered how tired you'd have to be to hand your baby to a stranger so you could nap, the answer is mother-of-two tired—a terrifying level.

My father is drawn to the sweetness of babies for the same reason I idolize my grandfather and Phil's face goes goofy at the sight of a dog. There are few things in this world that are good all the way through. When we are in the presence of one, we are momentarily cleansed. We are reminded that there is a more nourishing place for our spirits to live. Like babies, we can delight in the whipping of fan blades or our own reflections. We can reside in the present moment. To be still with that wisdom, that innocence, is at once calming and energizing. It's the ultimate mindfulness.

It's the same reason my father likes prayer. As someone who suffers from joint degeneration, it forces him to concentrate on something other than his pain, and the way that pain has redirected his life. Holding a baby is like chanting a mantra—the edges of reality blur into the background. It centers him.

He leaves a comment on a friend's Facebook page, thanking her for bringing her baby to his house. He says it was the only time in the last few weeks he didn't hurt. It's difficult for any task to compete with screams that come from inside your joints, but perhaps the light of a baby was striking enough to interrupt that pain, to make it flinch long enough to say, Enough! Look at the swirl of feathery hair at that top of this infant's precious head, the way its lips work in sleep. I will not miss this.

The next thing my dad writes is, "Maybe if I have grandchildren, I'll finally be pain-free." He might as well have tagged me.

My sister-in-law's comments are more like prophecies. She staggers into the house with bag straps cutting off circulation in her forearms—enough gear to clothe and feed her kids for weeks rather than a weekend. She raises an eyebrow at me and says, "This will be you one day."

My mother-in-law's prods are earnest. "What is causing you to hesitate?" she asks. "Children are the greatest gift, the best thing you can do with your life. You won't regret it."

But I think mothers often regret it; they just aren't allowed to say so. And her insistence on the positives without mentioning the squawking, puke-stained negatives remind me that, if I'm unhappy as a mother, I'll have to keep it between me and my wine glass.

My mother is not so quiet about the struggle.

"I'm afraid I'll be miserable," I say.

"You will," she says. "Absolutely."

My mother is a pleasant person now. She talks to our family dogs in high-pitched voices and saves them bones from our dinner. She does Zumba videos in her underwear, and is tickled by bathroom humor. But I remember her incensed, hair braided tightly down her neck, lines carved between her eyebrows, her face pinched into a beak. For almost two decades, she traveled between degrees of exasperation, dusting with my father's holey socks pulled over her hands; scrubbing a bathtub, her back hunched, sweat glistening on her forehead; heaving a shovel into the earth, dirt streaking her cheek; dicing onions, garlic, carrots and butterflying chicken breasts for cutlets; carting us to this friend's house or that afterschool activity, gripping the steering wheel while glaring at the road ahead as if it was the reason her life had been reduced to this, taking bumps at such high speeds our asses floated above the seats.

She was our unpaid chef, gardener, cleaning lady, and shuttle service, menial work for a college-educated, licensed dental hygienist, all for the sake of three overweight children who were lazy and unappreciative of the cushy life in the suburbs she and my father had worked so hard to leave Queens and provide.

She attempted delegating, and paying us an allowance. She played good cop by painting our family as a commune, an intimate network that should share responsibilities. *Like hippies!* We didn't buy it. She guilted: *Leaving your crap there for me to put away implies my time is less valuable than yours.* She played bad cop by yelling, punishing, and yelling louder. She said ugly things. *This isn't the life I wanted. I wish I could take your father and run away.* We were afraid of her, afraid of the anger that hovered over our house. Her bad moods were storms, and we felt their electricity crackle in the air.

But we acted as if we were helpless to dissipate her anger, and even prevent it. We stared back at her dumbly from the couch. We said stupid things. *If you wanted help, why didn't you ask for it? I will, after the show. I don't know how to empty the garbage.* We made demands. *What's for dinner? I don't like that. I need to go to Amy's house. I don't want to ride my bike. I need new clothes. Jeans. But I don't like those jeans. Because they're old. No one wears jeans like that anymore. I don't want them from Goodwill or Bob's. I want them from American Eagle. Can I take voice lessons? But I hate the piano. Well, I didn't ask you to buy it. I didn't ask to be part of this family.*

With all her grief, how could my mother have been happy? In her position, could I be?

 ⬤ ⬤ ⬤ ⬤ ⬤

Wanting a baby is supposed to be my biological imperative, but I'm beginning to think my maternal clock ran out of batteries, or that the second hand snapped under the weight of hard cider and literary ambitions. Or maybe I'm like one of those rat moms from the famous study who just wasn't born with a nurturing gene, and Phil will be the parent responsible for licking our pups.

I'm afraid to have children. I'm afraid to birth a butternut squash and invite it to chew my nipples; to slip into sleepless insanity; to unknowingly apply poop mousse to my hair. I'm afraid of baby weight. I'm afraid of all the noise. I'm afraid because babies grow up to be teenagers, a lose-lose since teenage boys are smelly and teenage girls are mean.

I fear trading in my current identity for "mother." As a woman, I'm already at a disadvantage in a culture where "You aren't like other girls" is the highest compliment, where females are considered catty and not funny—heck, they don't even get the joke. (I could Stepford smile my way through being called catty, but if you undermine my sense of humor, I'll use my funny bone to impale you.) Women's interests are categorized and set apart in order to save men from having to bother with them: chick lit, romcom, women's fiction o,r even more cringey, *domestic* fiction. There's no men's fiction because male characters have ingrained mass appeal, while female characters and their relationships, outrages, heartbreaks, and injustices couldn't be of interest to those with a penis.

Mothers, the epitome of femaleness, are especially broken off from society. We expect them to raise their young and talk amongst themselves in kid-appropriate restaurants. We expect mothers to play their part, which means sacrificing everything else they are. They have to justify any time they are away from their family, even when they are working. No one sees a father and asks, "Hey, Steve, where are the kids?" because Steve is allowed to be more than one thing. He can have his job, his softball league, and his straight razor hot shave because he isn't just a dad, he's also an employee and an athlete and a human who grows a beard, and good for Steve, but it isn't equitable, because women are defined in total by their relation to their family. When we see Mrs. Steve So-and-So (and we can call her Mrs. Steve So-and-So) sipping beer with friends, we think, *Who granted this woman furlough?* Her pursuit of happiness is an indulgence, because any energy spent on her own interests is a direct deduction from energy she might have used to benefit her family. Therefore, she should always be in service, because she is Mother (and we'll critique how she's performing that role too). Dads can blow off steam—with their long day at the office, they've earned it—but if their wives get drunk, we make a franchise about it called *Bad Moms*.

· · · · ·

When I confess to my mother that I fear I'll be miserable as a parent, and she replies, "You will. Absolutely," she quickly adds, "But sometimes you won't be."

My mother is happiest now when she is with her children. She loves being a parent in the present tense, while she only enjoyed being a parent, past tense, sometimes. But if I ask her if it was worth the irritation, the madness, and the occasional despair, I know her answer will be yes.

Maybe in relationships, jobs, hobbies, pets, and children, the question should always be: does the good outweigh the bad? *You will be miserable. Absolutely. But sometimes you won't be.* More than wholehearted reassurances, this promise gives me hope.

Nothing is always good. The cost of joy is despair. Bliss means opening yourself up to outrage. Acquiring one end of the spectrum expands the whole breadth of your experiences.

There will be moments of outrage: fecal streaks down the wall, thrashing heads, yanked hair, spilled milk, tear streaks, bruises and scrapes, refusals, and time-outs. There will be playground disputes, bad grades, silent treatments, broken curfews, blatant lies and cunning ones, slammed doors, and angst. But there will also be pomegranate toes, pajama feet padding down the hall, storytime cuddles, inside jokes, and I love yous. There will be pillow forts, Disney sing-alongs, sun-kissed freckles, Santa lists, campfire s'mores, soccer goals, and first crushes. We'll create a person and watch him grow—and maybe even one day create people of his own.

I can't stuff the baby back in if I change my mind down the road, but I also can't snap a family into existence if Phil and I find ourselves longing for the divine chaos of family, the kind of company who triggers heartache that is outweighed only by their feverish devotion.

Regret over having a child might mean frustration, compromised independence, and a shift in identity, but regret over *not* having a child is a gutting absence, the nonexistence of life and how that life might have enriched you and those around you. I'd rather bear the weight of what is than what isn't, tolerate someone than suffer the blaring offbeat of their silence, be burdened by the heft of what I have than be haunted by the ghosts of the missing.

So we'll try, as they say, but it's the "try" of people who RSVP to parties with, "We'll try to stop by," which really means if they happen to show up, it'll be almost entirely by accident.

Before a baby materializes, I hope I'll swell with that mythical want women talk about. Sometimes I think I feel it when a wee one totters around and hugs strangers for no reason. There's an inkling that I've overlooked something, like that gnawing suspicion on the way to the airport that you forgot an important item at home. It passes through me like a spirit from another world. Then, in a flash, it vanishes. But it's possible that spirit will linger longer and longer until it finally settles down.

Letter to My Husband

Dear Bub,

We both know I'm not a modest sick person. I barf like I'm a bellowing walrus, and then sob like I'm sure the next heave will kill me. This doesn't bode well for pregnancy, so allow me to apologize now, because I won't later.

I hope you won't tire of simmering soup, ferrying water, and rubbing my stomach, which you claim doesn't do a thing but you're wrong because it definitely does. I hope you won't get annoyed by the sitcoms I watch on repeat in an unshowered ball of estrogen and sweat on the couch. But more than anything, I hope you'll remember, no matter how frustrated you feel, no matter how high-maintenance I become, you can't complain. Nobody will stretch your pee hole into an opening large enough to squeeze out a softball, so you best stroke my hair until your fingers freeze into an arthritic claw, and then you better switch hands.

I am nervous for how this experience will transform and possess me. I'm sure you are too, although you'd never admit it. Remember when we asked someone if he was looking forward to his baby, due in a week, and he replied, "I'm looking forward to getting my wife back"? The idea that I may disappear from your world, and from mine, is disturbing. Especially since, if I go, I won't be returning as the wife you knew. I'll be reshaped literally and figuratively, and if sympathy eating is real, so will you. You'll be Father. I'll be Mother. What will that do to us? There is no telling.

Most divorced couples have children. This includes our colleague who swears *his marriage fell apart because of sleep deprivation, and believes most couples would eventually reconcile if they could just slog through the first six years of their kids' lives. (I don't want to slog! I want to relish!) I'm sure kids are worth whatever consequences the stress of their care brings, but I don't know our children yet. I only know us. We are gambling our happiness. We're in for a big payoff if we win, but there's so much to lose.*

There are also forces outside us that can have an effect and be affected. Will Penny be aggressive to the baby, forcing us to make a decision that will break our hearts? Will our parents clobber us with their presence, our lives suddenly becoming theirs to share, dividing us into too-small pieces? Will our friends still invite us over if we're lugging a diaper bag, or if the untrained two-foot chimp we bring shoves everything in his mouth and poops on their throw pillow? How long before we are left out of plans?

You would ask the last question with a happy upturn at the end. I can hear you now, offering to watch the baby, encouraging me to go on without you. And I will, but I don't want to make that a habit; I don't want to go on without you.

Promise to come with me wherever we may go (and bring Penny).

Bub

PART II

First Trimester

On Losing Someone You Weren't Sure You Wanted

Take One: Five Weeks

My period is late.

An Internet search suggests that the flu can have that effect, and I do have some sniffles, so I'm convinced for five days. On the sixth day, doubt rattles my confidence. I take a pregnancy test purchased in bulk on Amazon—ten tests for six dollars. The deal would have sounded sketchy, but the seller's name was Blue Cross, which is medical, and the product was rated four stars by a thousand reviewers.

It's negative.

Over a beer the following evening, I pitch my flu theory to my friend Andrea, a physician assistant, expecting confirmation. (I am sick enough to dry out my period but apparently not enough to sip an IPA.) She's never heard of such a thing.

"No kidding," I say, and order another beer, because the test was negative.

I teach class—no period. Tulip stalks break through the soil—no period. The world's oldest person dies after 117 years—and that's how long it's been since I've seen my dear Aunt Flo. On day eight, I take another discount pregnancy test. When it again presents one line rather than two, it occurs to me that maybe, just maybe, the tests are no good.

Upon further examination, I find that the majority of Amazon customers rated the test five stars, but 25 percent rated it one star because of the test's insensitivity at the early stages of pregnancy.

When else do you take a pregnancy test but in the early stages? What woman in her third trimester is reaching around her globe of an abdomen and then waddling over to her computer to submit her five-star rating?

Now that I realize my previous results were about as reliable as if I'd peed on a Q-tip, that I was swindled by a charlatan in Blue Cross clothing, I buy a three-pack of name-brand tests and pee on a thick, first-class stick with a thumb notch and everything. Turns out the extra $4.50 yields about as luxury an experience as you can get while crouching over a toilet, as well as another crucial accessory: an additional line. I drink two full glasses of water and pee again. Armed with a missing period and two positive tests, I am beginning to think I might be pregnant.

In my imaginings of this moment, my eyes stung with tears of joy. *A baby! We're going to have a baby!* Living it, though, I feel surprise more than anything. I stopped taking birth control five months ago, but we also tracked my ovulation and avoided days in which conception was likely. When the app reported above 8 percent, we metaphorically blew out the candles and paused the Al Green track and literally got out the Thai food leftovers. If you can call this "trying," then we were "trying."

I emerge from the bathroom, my eyes indeed glassy, but not with joy. "Well, I'm pregnant," I say to Phil and shrug. "Can we go to the beach?"

The ocean sparkles like rhinestones have been sewed to its surface and our shoes shift in sand. Penny pulls to greet a Saint Bernard puppy whose fur and edges are soft, not yet coarse and made hard by age.

It's a cool April evening, and the air feels even colder on the shore. We walk the length of this familiar retreat, back and forth, back and forth. The unconscious movement allows my brain to process more actively, and the crisp stillness provokes clarity. I am grieving life as I know it. Pregnancy and parenthood will alter the only me I've ever known, inevitably transforming me into someone I haven't yet met, and therefore don't know if I will like.

More trivially, but not altogether irrelevant, frequent pleasures have been made suddenly forbidden: no more post-workout wine with Andrea, and no second jolt of caffeine when the afternoon lull hits. I dread the inconvenience and suffering of debilitating nausea. (My fear of vomiting verges on an anxiety issue. Simply being in a situation in which puking would be inconvenient, like on the inside seat of a restaurant booth or at a Broadway show, makes me dry-heave.) Not to mention the sacrifices and challenges of becoming a parent. There is no denying it: our lives will never be the same.

When we return home, I delete the ovulation app from my phone (some good it did) and download a pregnancy app. I calculate my approximate due date, research milestones, and sort the coming year:

Peak morning sickness will hit after finals, I'll be five months along for our Montana trip, we can't go to Florida for Thanksgiving. I'm going to be huge at the end of the fall semester. A holiday delivery. Baby's first Christmas, right off the bat. I'll start the New Year as a mother.

I begin to plan, and find comfort in logistics.

The next morning, I wake on my side in—for lack of a better term—the fetal position. Penny ventures farther up the bed and plops down in the space between my knees and my chest. I drape an arm over her and realize she fills the space my belly will soon occupy, curled in the place and shape of my future child, whose cells are multiplying inside me at that moment. *There are four of us in this bed.*

At five weeks, the embryo is the size of an orange seed and has a tail. I picture it swimming around, flexing its mobility, getting acquainted with its new digs. I'm not overjoyed at the thought but, in the sleepy light of morning, spooning my dog, my husband snoring beyond her, the trees outside my window a silhouette against the coral sky of dawn, and the magnolia blossoms across the street just beginning to open, I feel something like peace.

My abdomen cramps an hour later. Toilet paper surfaces a deep red clump of floundered possibility, tissue on tissue. A clot the size of a seed is cradled by blood-orange discharge, like gory oyster innards clasping a pearl. The baby-to-be now would never.

I cry. This both surprises me and doesn't. Something—some*one*—inside me has died. I hadn't gotten used to the idea of this baby yet, but the possibility to become attached, to learn and to love someone new, was just ripped away. I think of who this person might have become had things gone differently: a poet, carpenter, nature lover, Red Sox fan. I mourn all the possibilities. I am the only person it ever knew, and this is its funeral.

I want a postmortem. Did I drink it to death? Was it stewing in a poisonous bath of Starbucks Pike Place brew and all the alcohol I consumed in the previous weeks, including the drinks I sipped when my period was late and I should have known better?

Or my real fear: did it sense my ambivalence? Maybe it had been excited to announce itself to me, and my brain sent a disappointment hormone to it like hate mail. I wasn't overjoyed by the positive pregnancy test, but I cry because what made it positive is now flushed down my toilet.

My gynecologist sends me for blood work. She warns I might have to return once a week for three weeks until they can confirm the pregnancy is lost. Until then, I might have to rest to give my body the chance to salvage the pregnancy. I dread that uncertainty and imagine my body fighting to save this embryo, attending to it like a team of paramedics, checking vitals, hooking it to IVs, shocking it with defibrillator paddles when things turn for the worst. I never knew the death of something so little could take so long.

It's one of the first warm days of spring, the kind that inspires premature flip-flops and women to shave their legs, maybe even above the knee. Outside, the sky is dramatically blue and streaked with wisps of clouds. Inside, I am bleeding. But I have to go to work. I can't stay home for five days, hibernating in my cave like a prehistoric woman.

I discuss elements of fiction in front of my classroom while my uterus pumps out the furnishings its most recent occupant left behind. I lecture about indirect character development while blood clots collect on the pad in my underwear. My students listen, or they don't, while I try not to dwell on the tissue I am passing. It feels like someone is wringing out my organ. Sometimes the discomfort is so loud it's hard to hear a student's question.

My doctor calls to report the tests are conclusive: I've had an early miscarriage after what is called a chemical pregnancy. To my ears, the term seems to qualify the pregnancy, to suggest it wasn't legitimate. Only a *chemical* pregnancy, not as real or as valid as others. But really the name refers to the single way that early pregnancy can be diagnosed when the embryo is too small to be found on an ultrasound, by chemically testing for the pregnancy hormone hCG.

The most common cause of a chemical pregnancy miscarriage is a chromosomal abnormality that makes the embryo unviable from the get-go. Basically, my body likely knew it couldn't work and ejected it. It wasn't my fault.

Still, I ask the nurse, "Was it because I drank? Doctors often recommend not to drink if you are even trying to have a baby."

That gracious lovely angel on the other end says, "Honestly, dear, I tell women to live normally until they know for sure. It could take a long time to get pregnant. What are you going to do? Enter a monastery? These things happen. It wasn't because you drank."

Experts estimate that up to 75 percent of pregnancies end in miscarriage. Often women don't even recognize what's happening to them; they assume the cramping and discharge is just a severe period—that's how accustomed we are to enduring pain—and power through it without further investigation. Other times, we do know.

● ● ● ● ●

The standard recommendation is to wait to reveal pregnancy until the second trimester to reduce the likelihood that a formerly pregnant woman has to disclose her miscarriage. This guideline has particular merit in the age of social media, when pregnancy announcements come in the form of ultrasounds and baby shoes artfully arranged atop a pallet wood sign, or mom and dad posing in a meadow, and are dissem-inated to a couple's eight hundred closest friends. It would be upsetting to follow that manicured fanfare with a grim status update. But the advised timeline inadvertently suggests to women that anything that occurs before thirteen weeks should remain a permanent secret—that grief-stricken mothers shouldn't burden anybody with their loss. They have to mourn alone. (Or, as is my case, with a husband who offers the most emotionally complex consolation he is capable of: a panicked stare.)

Phil tells nobody. That's his way. I tell everybody. Sharing is my processing mechanism. Just as I peel back layers of a novel and make new connections each time I discuss it in class, I become an expert of my own experiences only after I've relived them beat by beat. I also observe and absorb the reactions of my audience, amassing multiple interpretations, and only when I see another's remorse or hear their voice can I determine if they are reflecting my own feelings back to me. Only when I detect something familiar can I put a name to my own pain. Learning the world and myself kind of like a baby does, I suppose.

· · · · ·

My abdomen has calmed. The cramping has faded into painlessness. It's over. There's finality in that—reverence and grief too.

I think of women who so desperately want a baby, who finally get that second pink line they've been praying for, and then experience that telltale ache above their pelvis. I think of those who have to wait three weeks until they know if their body failed to save the dream lan-guishing inside them. I think of women in the midst of miscarriage who go on with the daily tasks of their lives: pumping gas, sitting in meetings, consulting with clients, maybe speaking into the phone at the doctor's office, telling other women they are sorry for their loss. I think of those further along, whose babies have matured from orange seed to orange, who suffered symptoms of pregnancy, who grew attached to a new reality and got to know the life at their core.

I can only imagine their devastation, because although I was "trying" for this baby, they were meager attempts. Still, I know I'll be thinking of that baby-to-be throughout the markers of the coming year, when I don't have morning sickness, when my belly fails to expand. I'll be missing my baby this holiday season.

You Make Me Sick

Take Two: Eight Weeks

THE DOCTOR ADVISES WE DON'T HAVE UNPROTECTED SEX UNTIL MY NEXT period to allow my uterine wall to rebuild. After ten years together, Phil and I aren't desperate enough to drive to the pharmacy, stand in line, and buy a pack of condoms for the first time since college, all to use one or two and toss the rest in my bedside table behind my mouth guard. We are satisfied watching an extra episode of *New Girl* in hot chocolate–stained pajamas. That is until four days before my next scheduled period, when we have a glass of wine and figure a single time is just one away from a virgin birth. What are the odds?

My period never arrives.

According to online forums, it is common to completely skip a month of menstruation after a miscarriage. The uterine wall is rebuilding, and construction projects always take double a contractor's estimation. When you think of it that way, it really makes sense that it would be two months before my next cycle. It'd almost be strange to *have* a period. (I should add Justifying Missed Periods to the special skill section of my resume.)

· · · · ·

Peony buds burst into great handfuls of lush petals. Sweaters are packed away for the season. Phil and I, both college instructors, submit our final grades and flee for the Canadian border.

Through our tour of Quebec City and the neighboring countryside, my breasts are tender and my bras fit tight. I unleash my boobs from their prisons and cup them in my hands in hotel rooms. I chalk the sensitivity up to my body readjusting after the miscarriage, or maybe a second round of puberty. I always wanted to be a couple inches taller, and at least puberty would explain why I still get zits in my thirties.

Soon the chocolate croissants settle crossly, and the goat cheese gets goatier. I feel so yuck we drive home early. When the symptoms remain days after our last poutine, I take another a pregnancy test.

With the previous pregnancy, the line reddened so faintly we had to squint at it. Now it pops like a firework. I pee on three more sticks, and we have our own little Fourth of July.

Since Phil and I had sex once—*once*—I debate calling the hospital right then and there to book a stay, nine months in advance; I have a feeling there will be no room at the inn.

• • • • •

Pregnancy sends a woman's body into a tizzy from the start, propelling menstruation hormones into overdrive. It's as if your period had a nervous breakdown, went to Vegas, snorted a line off a stripper, and got pregnant. Progesterone and estrogen spike, prolactin levels skyrocket to twenty times the norm, relaxin to ten times, cortisol to a modest three, and a brand-new hormone is added to the cocktail. hCG doubles every *two days* throughout the first trimester. In addition, the body pumps out four pounds of extra blood. It's a mess of fluid, proliferating cells, and chemicals, and this pandemonium makes itself heard, seen, and smelled.

Two months pregnant, my boobs feel like a couple of prizefighters, swollen, heavy, and purpled in their preparation to breastfeed. I'm all for planning ahead. I arrive everywhere fifteen minutes early, and start considering my next vacation at the tail end of my current one. But these bruised speed bags are making moves to produce milk seven months out, which seems excessive, even to me.

I don't know if it's the prenatal vitamins, hormones, or change in diet, but the bathroom is suddenly a training ground for labor and delivery. When I don't have constipation, it's the opposite. Unsure if this is normal, I find myself in one of the many online pregnancy forums, where women speak in so many abbreviations, it's as if they're being monitored, but by an unsophisticated group just out of code-breaking school. One woman writes, "I was constipated when I was pregnant with my DS (dear son). BTDT. (Been there, done that.) Now that I'm pregnant with my DD (dear daughter), I'm thinking, TGID (Thank God it's diarrhea)!'"

Thank God it's diarrhea. That's my life now.

Sore breasts and bowel irregularity are nothing, though, compared to morning sickness, which is an insultingly minimizing term. When you are incapacitated all the livelong day, it isn't morning sickness, it's just sickness.

I never feel good, just varying degrees of unwell. Sometimes I feel like a bike pump is perpetually bloating my belly. Though there are . . . ahem, occasional leaks . . . the air supply is infinite. Sometimes I feel good old-fashioned queasy, like I'm recovering from a bender or ate a heap of fried clams. And sometimes I feel like I have a full-on stomach bug. I lurch to the toilet and spew like I'm the girl from *The Exorcist* and the baby is my demon.

Brushing my teeth, flossing, even too big a yawn triggers dry-heaving. Swallowing a pill makes me full-out barf, so when I have a headache, I nibble six oversize tablets of children's Tylenol, bit by sweet sandy bit, or I choke down four liquid servings, sucking the syringe like a baby lamb.

After all my worry that I'd miss coffee, wine, beer, sushi, and cold cuts, the only thing I can stomach is water and the edge of a burnt English muffin. Untoasted bread, the laptop screen, tissues—everything is stinky and rotten and terrible, and I just wish to be left in a ball on the couch to decay. Pregnancy is the world's longest road trip, and I'm carsick with months to go.

Often it takes a great deal of willpower and an intentional pause for me to convince a round of vomit to stay in my stomach. I can't even bring myself to speak, because each word has the physical weight of a marble, and my tongue working through a sentence would be as repellent as stuffing my face full of glass spheres. I gag just thinking about it. At least I'm enduring this over the summer, when fruit is in season (bless all the watermelons) and I teach online classes. If I had to stand in front of a room of students, it would not be words of wisdom I'd spew.

I can't write. Characters need my help getting out of trouble, but the light of the computer is gross. Thinking is gross. This is what makes pregnancy nausea distinct from other sickness I've experienced: even abstractions are repulsive. Any sort of stimulation, or even thinking about stimulation, is as activating as the stench of eggs, so there aren't enough saltines in the world to get me through a scene.

It's always bad, but I never know when it's going to be really bad. Can we go to our friend's barbecue, or am I going to puke in their bushes? Can we stroll the Gloucester waterfront, or am I going to puke at the feet of the fisherman statue? Can we visit my brothers in Boston, or am I going to puke in the Charles, a possible improvement to the water quality?

Perhaps the most difficult part is that I've developed an aversion to dogs. The house reeks of an animal den. It's in the couches, the rug, our bed. I can't escape it. The stench crawls into my nose and wakes me up at night. We are dog-sitting my brother's border collie, and she smells like a shoal of shrimp croaked in her mouth. Her fur evokes a towel that's been in someone's damp cellar—not basement, *cellar*.

Phil washes the wood floors with water and vinegar. He dusts the carpets and couch with baking powder and vacuums it up. We buy enzyme solutions designed to attack the source and deodorize. The smell still slaps me across the face when I enter the house and sits on my chest until I leave.

My friend's vision was compromised as a child, and he remembers putting on glasses for the first time and realizing with shock and awe that the trees were topped with individual leaves rather than a bushy haze. I feel like I'm experiencing the same epiphany, but with my sense of smell. A veil has been lifted from my nose, and I'm suddenly sniffing odors I assume everybody else has observed all along. I send apology texts to everybody who has ever visited. *I'm sorry for what you may have smelled when you had dinner here the night of March 15, 2017. I had no idea.*

Penny notices that I'm less affectionate. She follows me around the house and plops at my feet. We've converted our guest room (what will eventually be a nursery for the puke monster) into a clean room. I go there when I need to escape the animal I love but suddenly can't stand.

I am at my body's mercy, and the summer is passing me by. The season of wading into the frosty Atlantic Ocean, kayaking in the fingers of salt marshes (salt marshes—blek!), admiring sailboats bobbing in the harbor, sipping sangria on patios, and cracking lobsters (lobster—double blek!!) is happening without me. The very idea of humidity makes me want to barf, so I hole up inside my house with the air-conditioning at its highest setting.

Wed or unwed, babies are little bastards.

The nausea has lasted so long now, every day for five weeks and counting, sometimes I can't remember what being well feels like. Maybe this is how it has always been. I can't peer through the sick fog to see into the past. Maybe I've always been miserable.

Other women speak about turning inward at this time, submitting to the wonder of their bodies and this new little being they are creating. The hum of the outside world fades into the background as they sit still and listen to their private rhythms. They graze their tummies with painted fingertips and nap inside a sunbeam atop a quilt that's been handed down through generations. They are sleepy and thoughtful and content. I'm sweaty. While they sip tea, take quiet walks, and meditate on their divine capabilities, the work their body has set out to do, I spoon my toilet wearing only underwear and moan. Some pregnancies are so magical women commemorate them with photo shoots, donning flowing dresses and flower wreaths as they wade into their local stream. Capturing my experience would make about as much sense as inviting a photographer to document food poisoning.

Yet morning sickness isn't marketed as an excuse legitimate enough to opt out of obligations. Call out of work if you have a stomach virus, but an expectant mother better get her ever-growing ass in her seat. And if someone with a bug stays home from a family weekend, it's the right choice. They should rest, and we certainly don't want them to spread it around. But if I stay home because pregnancy is making me feel nasty, I can imagine the eye rolls. *Does she think she's the first pregnant woman in history? Other women suck it up. Why can't she?* People don't care if you're sick as long they can't catch it.

Women's bodies are abducted by alien life-forms, but we demand that they go about their day as normal. My friend had severe morning sickness and commuted an hour on the train, snacked on pieces of cereal throughout the day to try to keep her nausea at bay, commuted home an hour, and barely stepped off the train before she upchucked at the station. This happened every day for three months before nausea was swapped for knife-stabbing heartburn. (Heartburn—it's nice having something to look forward to.)

How can we claim women are more sensitive when our biology compels us to tolerate so much? And why must we tolerate it in the first place?

It's hard to believe we've put humans on the moon but haven't figured out an effective treatment for morning sickness. Today's remedies are shite. I've tried them all. I chew crackers before bed, and then first thing in the morning. I eat small meals periodically. I've taken Tums, ginger tea, and Alka-Seltzer. Nothing works. Nausea coats everything with the residue of a too-sticky adhesive that's impossible to remove. I'm alone in the antique house of my body while the world continues without me on the other side of grimy windowpanes. If we'd had better representation in the STEM disciplines all along, some she-nius would have solved our problem by now.

Pregnancy is a nine-month buffet of chronic illnesses: irritable bowel syndrome, acid reflux, constipation, fatigue, sleep apnea, vaginal varicose veins, acne, hemorrhoids, diabetes, obesity, urinary tract infection, insomnia, gingivitis, and vertigo. Nausea is the first course; I've only just begun.

I think of the single pregnant women who don't have a partner to bring them tepid water. I think of pregnant women with children who have to worry about keeping other humans alive when it's hard enough staying upright. I think of pregnant women who work in the food services—friends, they are the real heroes.

I always thought I'd dread the birth, the impending pain, the way it might change my body irrevocably. But now I see it as my Independence Day. A true delivery. The day I free myself of an invader, like Will Smith barreling out of the mother ship. It ain't over until this fat lady sings.

While I'm miserable, I'm accepting congratulations. I never understood why people offer congratulations at the beginning of something, like getting married or having a baby. People have been getting knocked up since the beginning of time. For many, it happens by accident, or, as in my case, more quickly than you hoped. It's different if conceiving wasn't easy. Then, by all means, congratulations! But for me, congratulations feel undeserved. Congratulate me when I've struggled through something, like after I manage to contract a seven-pound sack of bones and blood from my vagina, or once we've survived the sleepless stage. Congratulate me if we raise a kid who isn't an asshole in the grocery store. For now, you're just saying, "Congratulations, you're going to feel like shit for a really long time," when what you really should be saying is, "Hang in there," or "Good luck," or "It sucks, but most people think it's worth it in the end."

Ah, the end. It comes with a baby, which I still can't fathom, but it also means consuming a meal that wasn't purchased from the snack aisle, wanting a cup of coffee, leaving the house without a barf bag, speaking without heaving, burying my face in Penny's fur without consequence, smiling unrestrained, writing, thinking, living with the vibrancy that comes with feeling *good*, and appreciating the world again, with all its flavors, loud sounds, and vivid colors.

When this pregnancy is over, as God as my witness, I'll never eat another rice cake again.

First Look

Ten Weeks

THE WAITING ROOM IS OCCUPIED BY CUTE BUMPS BENEATH SUNDRESSES and round drums whose wait won't be long. My own belly is hard along the uterus, but not protruding, or at least not more than usual. These women offer glimpses of who I may become, after the feeling rotten stage is behind me. Maybe I'll be the glamorous Latina with thick, cascading hair and Jackie O sunglasses. Maybe I'll be the gentle blonde balancing a book on her perfect pregnant belly. Then a giant lady busts through the door, as miserable as this sweltering July day, tall and wide with thick limbs and a belly so inflated she has to rotate her body with each step, like the Stay Puft Marshmallow Man tramping across Manhattan, and I know in my heart that she is me.

A nurse calls my name and shepherds Phil and me to an exam room. She is middle-aged, has limp, ashy hair and a mouth set in a permanent scowl. She's the type to vacation in Atlantic City, parking herself at a slot machine with a watered-down whiskey sour and nowhere else to be.

She asks me to step on the scale before I change from my clothes into the wispy, weightless gown, which I find to be RUDE. I kick off my sandals.

"How much do you think those weigh?" she asks.

I untie my cloth belt and yank it from my shorts.

Since I haven't been able to eat in over a month, I've lost a bit of weight—four whole pounds, in fact. That drops me to 150.5, which is borderline on the doctor's scale, prompting a painful weighing experience.

The nurse shifts the large weight from 0 to 100, and when the balance drops heavily to indicate how far from 100 I am, she throws the javelin of the small weight. It skids from 0 to 50 pounds, and when it hits the other end, the balance still hasn't budged. She then has to shift the heavy weight to 150, and inch the small weight back tick by tick.

"Imagine if you still had your flip-flops on," she says.

To treat my morning sickness, she recommends 50 milligrams of vitamin B6 three times a day, half a tab of Unisom at night to deplete the secretions that cause nausea, and pure ginger tablets. Not ginger hard candies, which contain sugar that could aggravate nausea. Ginger tablets. Eating small amounts of protein every few hours: nuts, hummus, peanut butter. Staying away from carbs. They imitate relief at first, but then something about insulin and blood sugar ultimately makes you feel worse.

She issues this list as if they are greatest hits we're all tired of hearing, but they aren't suggestions I found in articles with titles like "10 Ways to Fight Morning Sickness," "How to Show Morning Sickness Who's Boss," and "Pregnant and Regretting Everything?"

Doctors wait to see an expectant mother until ten weeks, which makes sense with the high rate of early miscarriage, but these suggestions sure would have been helpful five weeks ago, which in puking years is more like five hundred.

Phil sits rigid on a bench inside the undressing alcove, the curtain pulled open to reveal him, the lone specimen of testosterone in a gynecologist's office. He directs his attention to his clipboard, occupied by a clear task. *Man take notes.*

The nurse guides us to an office the size of a converted closet where the doctor is waiting behind her desk. She is a bulky grandmother who has been doing this so long and has accumulated such a wealth of information, it's been compacted into a memorized speech she delivers like a racetrack announcer.

The list of genetic testing whirls around our heads as a tornado of scary words, procedures, and statistics. Phil and I blink and nod. I think we request the tests. I'll know for sure if we get results.

"I see you've lost a couple pounds. That's okay, but you're going to have to increase your calorie intake," she says.

I've been aware of my weight since I was eight years old, when a pediatrician told me I was in the 50th percentile for height and the 80th for weight, and I asked, pitifully, "So I'm 30 percent overweight?" My first diet was in fourth grade and, since then, the only time approached skinny was when I went through a breakup in my early twenties. Even just four years ago, a doctor read my 150-pound weight and, without inquiring about my diet or exercise habits, suggested I lose twenty pounds. (I gained five, in protest.) I've NEVER been told to increase my calorie intake. My eyes water. Maybe I love this baby already.

After the doctor's monologue, there is time for questions, probably because she is winded.

I say, "We only had sex once after the miscarriage, so I really didn't think I was pregnant, and it was the end of the semester, so there were parties. I did a bit of drinking."

She waves the concern away. "Put it out of your mind. The baby is fine."

I stare at my feet. "Like five drinks a week," I say, although it was more like ten.

"It doesn't matter."

Over the weekend, a pregnant friend reassured me, confessing that she still has a glass of wine with dinner. At hearing the doctor's insistences, I wonder if she is of a similar mind. I ask, "In that case, is it okay to still have a drink once in a while?"

She jerks her head. "No."

"Not even a glass of wine with dinner?"

"Not a drop."

It can't be simultaneously true that my previous drinking was absolutely fine but any future drinking is strictly forbidden. This nags me, and I want clarification, or really, a better explanation, but I've heard enough to know that this woman isn't the source for it. Perhaps she's seen too many horrors to allow for nuance, or perhaps she thinks providing patients with the full picture opens herself up to liability. Perhaps she doesn't want to risk being misunderstood, or having patients zero in on the wrong detail. Whatever the case, I know right then that I will search for the complex truth outside this office. In the meantime, I'll let my little bugger detox.

"Can I still exercise?" I ask.

The doctor is emphatic. "Of course. You can do anything you were doing before. Just, if you sweat, stop and hydrate. If you are doing a spin class, you begin to sweat, and everybody stands up, stay seated. Basically, if you're sweating, slow down." I'm half Italian—sometimes I sweat if a conversation gets heated. But there's more, so I don't interrupt. "Make sure you are never breathing so hard you can't talk through it. And if you're lying on your back, raise your pelvis so your blood pressure doesn't drop. And not a lot of work on your stomach. And don't fall. You'll be surprised how quickly your coordination and balance gets thrown, and you can't fall, so be careful. Other than that, you're fine."

As far as exercise goes, this leaves grocery shopping. Phil scribbles furiously.

I say, "We are going to Montana in a few weeks. It's a hiking trip."

"Hiking through a meadow?" she asks, hopefully.

"More like a mountain."

"Like I said, don't fall, don't sweat, don't let your breathing get too labored, and whatever you do, don't fall."

"Montana is famous for hot springs. Can I—"

"No."

"Not even if I only—"

"No."

Even before the examination, I feel bound to a table, each restriction and prohibition tightening the straps, all the eyes drifting toward my belly. My identity is blurring, melding to the fetus's, or reassigning to it completely. I can resist. I can fight the restraints and demand freedom. But I've entered a new reality where I don't bear the consequences of my actions alone. So I have a choice: I can insist on independence, behave as I see fit, or I can be a good mother.

The doctor exits and, in what is probably the least sexy disrobing Phil has ever witnessed, I wriggle into the gown.

When the doctor returns, she peels down the top to expose my breast. "Do you plan to breastfeed?"

"Yes."

The clinical style of her nipple tweak takes the tit out of titillation. "You have flat nipples, maybe even a little inverted. At thirty-five weeks, pinch them regularly like this. See how they are standing up now? It'll make breastfeeding easier."

I experience the psychological equivalent of the expression babies make when they lick lemons. I think, *Wait, wait, wait a second. These aren't normal nipples? What do other women's look like? How have I reached my thirties without ever knowing my boobs are weird? What else is different about me?* I'm suddenly dreading the pelvic exam.

While I'm wrestling an existential crisis, Phil, who perhaps was always aware of my chest aberration and said nothing, remains a fastidious student, watching the doctor's technique and scratching his pencil against his notepad. I imagine I'll later read, "Thirty-five weeks: pinch nipples," perhaps accompanied by a furiously rendered diagram of my apparently flat-as-sliver-dollar-pancake nipples.

The doctor squirts jelly on my belly with the delicacy of a carnie mustarding a hot dog, grabs a machine that resembles an oversize flip phone, and directs me to hold and position it so we both can see. Then she guides the wand across my abdomen.

"There's your baby. See its heart beating? See its little arm things? It looks good."

I concentrate to make sense of her screen, this detached window into the goings-on of my womb. I want to greet this human shape who has newly graduated from embryo to fetus, as big as a prune now, they say, with teeth budding below its gums, working kidneys, and developing bones—this being that will one day be my child, or already is my child, but one day I'll know and fiercely love as my son or daughter. Here is the reason I've been sick. Here is the reason everything has changed, and will never be the same. Here, should be, my life's most precious miracle. I wait for my synapses to detonate a Boston Pops Fireworks Spectacular of joy and maternal devotion.

The picture is coming into focus just as the doctor snaps her phone shut and wipes the gel off my stomach. The moment is gone. That was it. It wasn't a movie scene where Mom and Dad get a long emotional moment to hold hands, meet their baby for the first time, and fall hopelessly in love. I didn't hear a heartbeat. I didn't get a sonogram to take home, tape to the fridge, and contemplate. But I saw it, whoever it is. And it wasn't like that scene in *Friends*, when Rachel can't identify the figure. It may only be the size of a dehydrated plum, but technology has advanced enough that it actually resembled a baby. There was a head, and its heart lit up with every beat, and the doctor was right: it did have little arm things that flapped like it was splashing around in my stomach. Was that a hint of personality? Will this kid be jubilant?

It was only a flash, but Phil and I glimpsed our child for the first time. There's an extra heart beneath my heart. There's life in the little chapel of my womb, and it will grow and grow, forcing me to change and reconstruct with it. Then my holy place will be vacated and that celebrant will be in my arms.

I didn't cry or fall in love but, with this bit of tangible proof, I am beginning to believe in the magnitude of this unconscious act: building a new person, and deepening the individuals Phil and I are. My quality of life may be compromised, but perhaps that's the price of creation. I have to hold what pregnancy precludes me from doing against this tremendous feat. Our adventures are being curtailed, but for the sake of our most intrepid undertaking yet.

Letter to My Changing Body

Twelve and a Half Weeks

Dear Body,

They say pregnancy is a miracle, and they're right. I'm starving myself, yet my body is expanding. That's pretty damn miraculous.

In other words, lady, you're getting fat.

My rational brain knew you'd gain weight. It even knew the appropriate amount—between twenty-five and thirty-five pounds. Yet I'm frustrated by numbers ticking up on the scale. At nearly thirteen weeks, you don't look pregnant, exactly. There isn't a discernible bulge. I'd prefer the cute mama-to-be look found on Instagram under #babybump and #preggo, where women strategically place their hands to highlight the miniature basketballs that are already obvious under fitted maternity dresses. Although I can see how referring to a pregnant woman as "cute" can be patronizing—it desexualizes her and undermines her intelligence—dammit, I'd trade demeaned and cute for this. I just look like I've let myself go. I don't look #preggo, I look #IGaveUp.

My pregnancy app says the baby is the size of a peapod, but it doesn't look like I've eaten a peapod. It looks like I've eaten potato chips. And ice cream. And guess what—I have. Because I'm pregnant, and all I ate for ten weeks were saltines and watermelon, and I have about an hour every day where I can stomach something else. That hour is the food version of The Purge, in which I commit crimes against my stomach. Then, when the metaphoric hour is over, I literally purge.

Yesterday, a pair of pants that fit at the beginning of the day was tight by the end of the day. You, Body, are inflating like a balloon. When I go back to school in the fall, I imagine my students will watch it happening at the front of their classroom like watching the gum chewer blow up at Willy Wonka's factory. It's one way to get them to look up from their phones.

There's so much happening without my permission or cognizance, without my even trying. I study you in the reflection of a full-length mirror with, not quite wonder and not quite repulsion, but something like fascination. Look how I am evolving. Or, on less generous days, I'm a monstrosity.

Sports bras reshape my breasts, and they maintain their new contours even when free of their sweaty containers. It's like my boobs are moldable sandbags. They too are enlarging; my old bras fit like yarmulkes.

My areolas are two puddles of coffee being drained of their cream—ironic since they'll soon start producing milk. But they aren't darkening consistently. The colors in my right nipple are swirling, and when they settle I hope they'll tell me my future (wait, maybe that's tea leaves), and freckles speckle all around the nipple, as if from a cup-of-joe spit-take.

In all the pregnancy literature and shared mommy anecdotes about physical changes, nobody ever mentioned belly hair. The follicles have sprung in a thin but even coat, like a puppy belly, as if the baby is building itself a thatched roof. Maybe, like my flat nipples, belly hair is another anomaly particular to me. I wonder what the sage nipple-tweaking doctor would recommend—probably shampoo.

Body, I'm trying to admire you for the beautiful, wondrous act you are performing but, damn, girl. Belly hair? We have a long road ahead. Get your house in order.

Me

PART III

Second Trimester

Big Sky Country Meets Big Me

Fifteen Weeks

MONTANA IS PROBABLY A STUNNING STATE: SNOWCAPPED PEAKS, DOUGLAS firs, glittering lakes, gurgling rivers, the majesty of bison, gray wolves, and grizzly bears. But in my memory, the entire dusty wasteland is coated in a sheen of sweat, vomit I choked back, and vomit I puked up. The natives somewhat arrogantly refer to Montana as "The Last Best Place." I'm afraid I left it a little worse.

We booked the trip before the nausea fog that's hovered for twelve weeks and counting. Back then, when I was hungry, I ate. Hell, I often ate when I wasn't hungry. That's how privileged I used to be. I had no sense that one day soon I'd be tossed into a pit of queasy despair I'd be too malnourished to claw my way out of. It's only when you're sick that you realize how tenuous your health is. And if you are fortunate enough to become healthy again, I imagine you forget the lesson as suddenly as you learned it.

I never appreciated that each day I woke up and felt good, I'd been handed a gift. I'd give so much for relief now, even if only for a couple hours, to lift the screen of upset and remember how bright and crisp the world looks unobstructed, to do nothing but sit and feel good— simple as that, except it's not simple at all; it's serenity.

Pregnancy nausea is a long and bleak winter. I don't know when this is going to end, which is as terrifying as it is despairing. The guiding principle suggests it will subside after twelve weeks (which, by the way, is a long time to be sick), but here I am at fifteen weeks and nausea is still here too. Some women vomit every day for five, six months—some until a month after the baby is *born*.

In the weeks leading up to my trip, I writhe on the couch in the position of the little devil parasite making me ill and fantasize about cancelling the journey. It's bad enough to feel miserable in my living room. How could I survive on a trail? I can't imagine moving, never mind increasing my heart rate, huffing, trekking a mountain. And how would I fare being cooped inside a tent, breathing my own exhalations, opening a cooler, picking dirt—or what I hope is dirt—from my boots, sharing restroom facilities, and balancing on a stump, because of course we are planning to camp for the first time in my godforsaken life?

Nausea would be a heft I'd have to carry all day, in addition to my backpack. It's wearying enough to feel sick all the time. How will I heave my ill ass up to a summit?

We don't have trip insurance, but there is another possibility—we could just not go, lose the thousand dollars spent on flights, and disappoint the friend we are visiting. With not a small amount of gratification, I imagine our aisle and middle seats remaining empty as the plane's engines churn. Then the very idea of churning engines makes my stomach lurch and I have to stop thinking about it.

But what if I miraculously recover? They say morning sickness ends after the first trimester. So far they are liars, but maybe I'm just having a slow start to recovery. If I cancel the trip and then suddenly feel better, I'll be twiddling my thumbs at home, having squandered the money and all the pleasures of the vacation and visiting our friend. I delay any decisions. Then, before I know it, I'm in an Uber on the way to the airport, gulping the swampy air of industrial Revere, Massachusetts, from the open window.

I make note of all the restrooms at Logan Airport. On the plane, I keep my airsickness bag on my lap and slip Phil's into my seat pocket as backup. Despite the warnings of the nurse, I suck ginger candies for the duration of the trip, but anybody who has ever sucked ginger candies know they do absolutely nothing to stave off pregnancy nausea—and they taste bad.

With all the jerks and judders, it'd be easy to conclude that the passengers of Delta flight 963 are joining the pilot on his first flight. I'm not a gastroenterologist, but I believe I am filled with vomit from my stomach up through my throat. The only things keeping me from spewing the ugly contents of my body are gritted teeth, venerable self-control, and an airplane wing and a prayer.

On finally landing in Missoula, I beeline to the bathroom, an upright posture keeping everything in place, drop my bag in the corner of the stall, and erupt for several minutes. When I emerge, Phil is cringing with equal parts disgust and pity. Apparently the entire airport was privy to the reverberation of my regurgitation. I am not a delicate puker by any means—it's more like I think the toilet is mostly deaf and I'm shouting so it'll hear me—but they should consider themselves lucky that my performance didn't take stage when we were enclosed in a steel tube. Imagine my *La bohème* with those acoustics.

Montana is experiencing a record-breaking, triple-digit heat wave. It's so hot the state is catching fire. Our friend, whom we are staying with before together venturing into Glacier National Park, doesn't have air-conditioning. There is no relief until the sun goes down. I lay a wet washcloth on my chest and wait for winter or death, whichever comes first.

I venture to Montana despite feeling incredibly ill, despite knowing I can't enjoy anything to the fullest because the world is dimmed by sickness, because I don't want to spend my last childless year on the couch. I feel the urge to do and see while we still can, to get out there and live. This is our chance for one more grand exploration before being anchored by diapers, bottles, nap schedules, and cranky moods that aren't mine.

So we go, we do. There are odors made rank by my expectant super sniffer: the bag of trash in our car as we leave no trace, our unwashed bodies after days of hiking, porta-potties in need of emptying, and food that is confined and warmed over days in our coolers. But there are also strolls through spruce forests, river tubing, farm stand cherries, craggy mountains, glacial lakes, campfires, mountain goats and marmots spotted at over six thousand feet elevation.

What I'll remember most vividly is spotting two black bear cubs on a deserted trail. They are cartoonishly cute, with their oversize ears and puppy lumbering. But there is the matter of their absent mama, likely nearby, looking on. Does she see that we aren't a threat, that we let her babies pass unharmed, or is she verging on attack, because mothers love hard, murderously hard? Pine trees, glacial streams, wild berries—all those small pleasures fall away beside matters of vital importance. That mama bear isn't worrying about the grand adventures of her past, or looking forward to her next leisurely woods stroll without the nag of her cubs. She's zeroing in on the risks to her very purpose, her essence. She's seeing red.

This ferocious love is the crux of what I'm trekking toward: that one day I won't perceive the baby inside me, now the size of a pear, its skeleton ossifying, as the dead end to my escapades, but as the beginning of everything, not as a hindrance to my well-being, but as my very being. The path to motherhood is long and winding. Right now I'm navigating a tricky bit, where it is hard to gather up any fondness for the very thing causing my misery. But I'm hopeful that I'll eventually arrive at a greener glen, and the craggy resentment will drop out of sight behind me.

On the literal trail in Montana, we make noise to encourage the cubs along. As we clap and stomp, I think, *Please don't kill me, Bear. If I'm dead, all this morning sickness, all this suffering, will have been for nothing. But you get it. You're a mama too.*

A Womb of One's Own

Nineteen Weeks

DURING THE MOST UNPRODUCTIVE MONTHS OF MY ADULT CAREER, WHEN looking at a computer screen makes me want to yak, when I drape my lousy body over a couch and damn Eve's curse to hell, when my body and soul both feel malnourished, my first novel is sold and—miraculously, thrillingly, absurdly—optioned for a television series. This, after a decade of writing memoirs, essays, novels, short stories, and poems; submitting to literary magazines, agents, and small presses; receiving hundreds—maybe thousands—of rejections; deciding to give up; rewriting manuscripts; and deciding to really give up this time; this, when I am indisposed, incapable of working at all, is when I tap the glass ceiling enough that it shatters around me.

Like a humpback whale, I surface periodically from my gray of sick to accept congratulatory phone calls and laugh or weep with well-wishers at the absurdity of this delightful turn, and at such an unexpected time. Or, as my grandfather puts it, "A baby, a book, and a television deal? You could walk through a rainstorm and not get wet."

Television takes so long to produce, I'll be lucky if I'm alive for the release of the final product, if it ever leaves the ground at all, but the book is set for publication on what will, according to the due date, be the baby's first birthday.

I endeavored for a decade to do the author thing, and then, figuring that was by all accounts a lost cause, turned ever so reluctantly, even begrudgingly, to the mother thing. Now I'll perform two labors of love in parallel. For everything there is a season: a time to be born, and a time to publish. For me, those seasons are colliding, and I'll birth a book and a baby simultaneously.

The next several months will be dedicated to transforming my body and my body of work, admiring sonograms and then cover art, debating baby names and then book titles, finessing my language as well as my baby's organs. Then, inside my baby's first year, I'll breast-feed, diaper, burp, soothe, bathe, pump, dress, and chase while my other baby is packaged, marketed, distributed, and reviewed. For one, the bindings will be set, the ink dried, and the character's journey complete, while there are still infinite ways the other's story can turn out. Both will be subjected to the world.

I may find donning two new identities conjointly—Mother and Author—to be as seamless as layering necklaces or as bulky as shoving legs into two pairs of pants, or I may be so bewildered I'll forget to wear pants at all. My eyes may split following the different directions of book and baby. I may lose sense of who I am inside so much new skin, or I may retreat, burrow to my core, and discover who I was and what I wanted all along.

I enter the murky unknown, teeming with possible delight and strain, one hand on my tummy and the other on my keyboard, my teeth clenched against my next wave of puke.

· · · · ·

To celebrate my career advancement and the waning of queasiness, which now plagues me only half the day and then withdraws until the next sunrise, I treat myself to a spa package—discounted, of course. The validation of my book deal was boundless, but its advance came in the very real fiscal shape of a roof replacement.

The woman painting my nails is the spa manager. With her accent, unencumbered volume, no-nonsense attitude, and hair dye to spare, she is a true daughter of Boston's North Shore. She likes to gab—we cover pregnancy, my job, and most of her childhood—and she seems unable to chat and paint simultaneously, so I spend an hour with my hand perched in hers like we are new lovers, her miniature paintbrush suspended inches above my fingernails.

Then I'm passed over to the massage therapist, who asks if I have any medical conditions. News of my pregnancy thrilled the manager, and since I'm still getting used to the idea of being pregnant and trying to be excited about it, I share, figuring if I practice enthusiasm and see it performed by my audience enough times, maybe I'll feel it authentically. If not, at least this stranger should have the common courtesy to flatter me, insisting she would never have guessed, despite my bloated figure.

But when I announce that I'm pregnant, she stiffens. "I can't work on a pregnant woman."

I deflate everywhere but my belly. "Oh."

"The chance for miscarriage is too high. I just—I won't do it."

"But I've read all the prenatal books and I've never heard of such a thing," I say.

"Well, I have." With that, she walks me to the front of the business as if escorting a troublemaker to the principal's office.

The manager asks how I'd like to pay for the package whose services I won't be using. I slide my credit card across the counter, holding back tears. I'm not an emotional person. If you don't count when characters cry on-screen and my eyes water automatically because I'm a sympathetic crier, I weep only a few times a year. I can't explain why this interaction upsets me, and so I feel foolish. On the drive home, though, that vague sense of silliness gives way to more concrete indignation.

There are terrible inequalities in the world: racism, homelessness, hunger. A white lady deprived of a massage doesn't exactly spike on the radar of social justice issues. But I feel I was unfairly dismissed, deemed incapable of making a choice for my baby or myself. I don't expect to join forces with the ACLU, but what happened still had the whiff of sexism (or maybe that's just my heightened sense of smell).

Americans are accustomed to making decisions on behalf of women's bodies. Like the nurse who filled out my intake form, not by asking a question, but saying, "I'm writing that you don't drink alcohol since you are pregnant." Travel companies decide at what point pregnant women can fly, Disney Cruises being the most conservative, prohibiting pregnant passengers beyond twenty-four weeks, even with a doctor's approval. We touch a pregnant belly without permission. We vote on whether a pregnant woman can terminate, and for how long she has that option.

We say, *Should you be carrying that, ordering that latte, sipping that beer? Should you even be in a sushi restaurant?* A pregnant friend was refused a Caesar salad at Panera because the employee was certain she wasn't supposed to eat cheese with a rind (inaccurate).

Pregnancy can make a woman feel special, imbued with a secret superpower. Or it can make her feel apart from the world, underwater, or like she's living an in-between life. No matter what she feels, hers is treated as a collective experience.

The baby belongs to the world. A pregnant woman is more vulnerable than ever before, exposed to the criticism of family, friends, acquaintances, and strangers, or forced to ask their permission or offer trigger warnings. *I'm going to order a decaf chai now, as long as that's okay with everybody in this Starbucks.*

As a pleaser, I am so aware of this potential for disapproval, I've turned into a closet beer sipper. I bobble my open purse and pitch it from our restaurant four-top just so our friend has to gather the spilled lip balm, pens, and trail mix (when you're pregnant, life is a hike—pack for it) while I sneak a sip of Phil's pint, savoring those yeasty pricks on my tongue. (Phil teases me later, claiming the baby is stumbling around, knocking into my uterine walls, gripping the umbilical cord for balance.) And that is with people I trust; I wouldn't dare drink in front of acquaintances. At a whiskey tasting, I make a big show of not participating—*I probably shouldn't even breathe these fumes lest my fetus ferments!*—in case anyone missed the fact of my not drinking.

There are so many activities made illicit by the cells multiplying in one's abdomen: hot tubs, high elevation, intense workouts, contact sports, horseback riding, deli meat, fish with mercury, soft cheeses, paint, ibuprofen, kitty litter, and sitting or standing for too long (you better get it just right!). We scare women into worrying one turkey sandwich, one bath drawn too hot, one pet of the cat will be the misstep that kills her child. *Is that spicy tuna roll worth the risk? You better stick to your herbal tea and vitamins.* Never mind that different countries advise against different foods, and Japanese women don't give up sushi. American women would only be granted permission if there was a prenatal Makimono, rich with folic acid and vitamin sea. (Sorry.)

Once home, I can't turn up any studies on the relationship between miscarriage and massage, but according to Google, this massage therapist isn't the only one to refuse service to a pregnant woman, despite a dearth of data. Uncorroborated suspicions abound in the age of the Internet, where anyone with forty dollars a month or access to a library can provide the world with his version of the facts.

Ironically, the book I'd brought to read at the spa was *Expecting Better,* in which economist Emily Oster reevaluates and challenges studies that result in inappropriate or unsubstantiated parameters for pregnant women. For instance, pregnant women are restricted to one cup of coffee, but she found that the upper limit is closer to three, and while most doctors say no amount of alcohol is considered safe, she found that one drink a day does not negatively affect the fetus. The discrepancies are often because studies haven't controlled for other variables, even ones that should have been obvious. Women who drank more coffee miscarried at a higher rate because they also happened to be older than the non-coffee-drinking population. In addition, women with healthy pregnancies naturally avoided coffee because they were nauseated, while women with nonviable pregnancies didn't feel as nauseated and were able to indulge in their morning latte. Coffee didn't *cause* the miscarriage; the nausea of a healthy pregnancy precluded the *coffee.*

As for alcohol, the behavioral problems detected in children of women who drank could also have been a result of the cocaine 45 percent of the study participants admitted to taking. (That isn't a joke.) Some studies compared drinkers to non-drinkers without differentiating between those who enjoyed an occasional glass of wine and those who went on the kind of benders even spring breakers would consider a little extra.

We accepted these studies, though careless, because we don't mind if women, and mothers in particular, have to abstain from pleasure. That is the price they must pay for the privilege of procreation. Or we don't present the entire, complicated truth because we don't trust women to conduct themselves appropriately, even if given proper guidelines. *If we tell women it's okay to have a drink a day, that'll turn into two drinks, or they'll call an entire bottle of wine a single drink.* (These are arguments I've heard verbatim—from medical professionals.) So instead of explaining the shades of safe behaviors, we infantilize women, as if to say, "You aren't allowed because I said so." I have a feeling those studies would have been more carefully evaluated if they centered on Viagra's relationship to alcohol or caffeine. Those results would have come with an iPhone app and a beard kit.

With limits that will pertain to men, we are specific and direct. Drinking and driving isn't a zero tolerance policy. We trust the wider population to moderate themselves before getting behind the wheel. But when it comes to pregnancy, a strictly female condition, it's easier to tell women *no* than to bother with details. Dangers are augmented and simplified—alcohol is *bad*, coffee is *bad*—without nuance. Never mind that there are safe parameters. Never mind that fetal alcohol syndrome is rare, even among alcoholics. This isn't about science. It's about being risk-averse, even puritanical, in protecting the almighty fetus, at the expense of its container—I mean, its mother. If we want to be really safe, perhaps no sexually active woman should ever be served a drink or massaged without a negative pregnancy test. You just never know, you know?

Or, if we are so worried about the welfare of babies, if we fear massaging a pregnant woman, treating her body to relief and—God forbid—pleasure in a time when she is experiencing discomfort, maybe we should conduct a proper study and do the research. Let's nail down the cause of pregnancy nausea and devise a treatment with the same kind of haste we rejected male birth control because it caused "nasty" side effects: mood swings, acne, and depression. (Sound familiar?)

There is so much we don't know about pregnancy, perhaps because most clinical trials are funded by a government largely populated by men who, consciously or unconsciously, don't support such research. Or maybe because we couldn't conduct certain studies at all since, up until January 2019, pregnant women were on a federal list of research subjects considered "vulnerable to coercion or undue influence," a list that included children and the mentally disabled. Until we do our due diligence, and perhaps even after, let's mind our business.

Unless, of course, you are willing to give me a massage. Then come over quick. I'll be the thick lady lying atop her soapbox, naked under the sheet.

Oh Boy

Twenty-One Weeks

PEOPLE ALWAYS SAY, "I DON'T CARE ABOUT THE SEX. I JUST WANT THE BABY to be healthy," and that is true for me too. Healthy—yeah, yeah, of course—and for it to be a girl.

I want to put my baby in a "Nasty Woman" onesie, gift her Amelia Earhart and Frida Kahlo Barbies, and clean dirt from under her fingernails after a morning spent digging for worms. I want my daughter's hand to shoot up in class. I want her to scrape her knees fighting for the soccer ball, get lost exploring the woods, and marvel over the workings of a baking soda volcano. I want to raise a curious, fierce little lady.

I am going to show her all I've learned about the world and make her strong in ways I am still learning to be strong. She won't try to impress boys with giggles and false naivety. She won't let a mechanic condescend to her. She will never apologize for her opinions, predilections, identity, or because her existence seems inconvenient to somebody else. (If she's ever pregnant, she won't leave a spa until she gets her damn prenatal massage.) She is going to shove off any person who touches her in a way she doesn't want to be touched, stand by her beliefs and tastes, and love herself as I love her. I am going to put thirty-two years of my own self-doubt to good use. I will teach her to be brave, speak up, and take risks, because this is a learned skill like anything else—just a skill that girls aren't expected to acquire.

Plus, we've selected a squad of standout girl names, and zero boy ones.

Alas, the ultrasound technician glides her wand over my ever-growing abdomen, announcing in semi-bored singsong (as if she announces genders every day), "Looks like a boy." She prints the proof. I can't figure out where she is looking, but apparently my baby has a penis.

Still, I've learned a little something (no slight to my son) about my baby. Whereas before he existed only as high-grade nausea that is petering with every passing week (although, at twenty-one weeks, not quickly enough), now I've discovered something real. He's a *him*. *He* has a penis. It's not much to go on, but it's something—enough that I feel his presence, which has been largely abstruse, solidifying. I might have experienced the same had the technician frozen a frame that indicated the baby would be an artist or an accountant or even that he'd like broccoli. Until now, the idea of Baby has been an abstraction, the snow static of a television without a signal, white noise in my abdomen. Now a shape is forming somewhere behind the blizzard, and that shape, apparently, is phallic.

At least a boy will likely never discover that my braids are messy and I don't know how to pick the right shade of lipstick. I won't have to yank Satan's silk up his thigh, or ask what he's wearing underneath his baggy sweatshirt. I won't have to explain why dressing as a French maid isn't appropriate for high school costume day. We'll sidestep the sometimes thorny relationship mothers have with their daughters, where they urge daughters to live the life they couldn't and then resent them for it.

I can aspire to contribute another boy to our barbed but glorious world who asks permission, listens, values the contributions of all his peers, is as interested in female protagonists as he is in male characters, and is brave enough to interrupt another person's insults, even if that person is his friend. I can buy a "Boys Will Be ~~Boys~~ Good Humans" onesie.

We celebrate news of our son with a blue-frosted cupcake. Phil accuses me—the person who wanted to raise a girl that defied

convention—of now being conformist, and he is right. But I want
mark the occasion, and I can't rightly ask the baker to top her delicac.
with a frosted shaft and balls, so I'm gender normative for the sake
of a cupcake.

We feast on butter and sugar and recount how I gasped when
the wand illuminated the screaming skeleton of a face, like our baby
was wearing a Day of the Dead mask, which, in October, was at least
seasonally appropriate; how I was tempted to toss out our scroll of
blobby and nondescript sonogram images, but that felt like being a
bad mother, so I stuffed it in my purse to throw out at home. But
most importantly, we debate what in the world we are going to name
this man-child.

Phil has nixed most of my suggestions. Back when we thought we
might have a girl, I came across a character in a book named Aurelie.
I suggested it out loud, rather triumphantly, like I'd stumbled upon
a winning lotto ticket. Phil said it sounded at best like a method for
taking pills and at worst like a sex act; Aurelie was destined to have a
sister named Anna-Lee.

We move on to boy options. Since this baby was with me when I
secured a book and television deal, and at Fenway Park when the Mets
beat the Red Sox 8–0, I suggest Felix, which means "lucky." Nope.
Conan gets the negatory even though it means "little wolf," because
he's also a barbarian and a quippy redheaded talk show host. Noah is
the "If you're a bird, I'm a bird" guy from *The Notebook*. ("Exactly!" I
say.) Theodore gets vetoed because it recalls a douchey student. (This
is a common challenge for college instructors—every good name has
a frat boy to crush it like an empty beer can.) Wilhem Dillon is too
adjacent to "wheeling and dealing."

That leaves us with, well, Baby Boy.

Whatever we choose could alter the direction of our son's life. We
could give him a name he'll share with other students, creating a tribe
of Brads, or an appellation people will mispronounce his entire life,
making him unique, or equally misunderstood. Some names sound
more approachable. Some are more likely to be hired. Some sound like

u'd want to plan your bachelor party. Others sound like

ɔ'd pick you up at the airport, or the neighbor you avoid

ɪes on about the invasive species in his vegetable garden.

ʞe my name's open and rolling nature, alternating consonants

vowels, and its ethnic ambiguity. I like that it's almost entirely

ɪne. I so strongly identified with my name, I refused to surrender

ɪt to marriage. To give up the set would be to shed an heirloom. By name, I mean first and last. My middle name is that dress in the back of the closet you never wore because it fit awkwardly and you actually thought you donated years ago, but there it is.

My older brother, Greg, hates his name. He finds the hard *g* repellant, and he's got one on either end. To demonstrate his point, he orates his name as if he's gargling. He's sure his life would have been better, easier, if only the *g* could have been soft, as in Geoffrey. If he were a Geoffrey, he'd always have a fire crackling and a snifter of brandy within reach.

Phil doesn't feel connected to his first name. He identifies more with our nickname of "Bub." Perhaps that's why he's choosing our son's with care. He wants to select a name to which he feels tethered. Maybe the notion of our child is as thin and unformed to him as it is to me, and he's waiting to hear a name that speaks to him, that reaches through the great divide of my uterine wall and says, *I am yours, and you are mine.*

Naming someone we've never met, without any sense of his persona or identity, seems an impossible task. Do we choose a name that sounds charismatic or reserved? Fierce or compassionate? Hard or soft? Will he be a bachelor party or an airport friend? Or God forbid—the annoying neighbor?

• • • • •

This is on my mind when we see a Queen cover band perform at a century-old theater in town. An unlikely collection of 1970s British rock fans is seated in the row before us: a group of ten-year-old boys.

They wear oversize T-shirts, basketball shorts, and unwashed hair an dance, sing, and fist-pump from the opening number to the encore They belt all the words. When the drums cut out after the ballad portion of "Bohemian Rhapsody," the boys freeze, and then bop in synchrony along with the rhythmic piano that transitions into the operatic movement. These are songs they *know*.

They were born in the time of Britney Spears's "Womanizer" and are the age when one awakens to pop hits while Drake's "God's Plan" tops the charts. Yet they are enamored by oldies dreamed up forty years before they were conceived, originally sold as records, at least four storage mediums removed from the technology of their era.

When I was their age, I tuned into what my culture suggested for me—NSYNC, Ricky Martin, Spice Girls. Not something entirely outside of my peer group. How did they discover such quirky interests so early in life?

I admire the surprising opinions of these tiny groupies, who found their niche against the odds. I wonder what their names are, and if they are fitting: if the Sams are easygoing and the Alexanders are the leaders, or if these boys are redefining the connotations, making their names their own.

I watch them rock with all their might while their chaperones sit quietly on the periphery, and I'm reminded that, although I'm deliberating over my son's name, I can't choose his passion or identity. If we had a girl, she wouldn't necessarily have turned out to be the one I'd envisioned, with grass-stained shin guards, an aversion to pink, and confidence to spare, and I wouldn't have had the right to expect her to defy stereotypes. Requiring an untraditional path is still casting her into a role. Likewise, I can't mandate the person my son will be. His passion might be eccentric and endearing, like loving music four decades out of date, or more mainstream, like lacrosse and Bruno Mars, but that is wonderful still, as long as it is his. His identity will be his own, and I shouldn't pressure him to conform. Maybe I'll have to put those messy braids to work after all. (Can I draw the line at stockings? I really hate stockings.) My job, in addition to keeping him

ng him from becoming another douchebag Theodore,
s interests, support, nurture, and encourage him to be his
r without shame.

ing the flouncy notes of "Bicycle Race," two pairs of
drinking Massholes swat the arm of one of the kid's parents, ges-
e emphatically toward the boys, and demand they sit down because
neir foot-stomping celebrations are blocking the view of fake Freddie
Mercury. I want to elbow those people in the throats (mama bear
instincts revving?), especially when one of the boys notices their
heckles and slumps self-consciously, half-dancing while still trying to
accommodate the jerks' line of sight.

If the music weren't blasting, I would urge that sweet boy to stand
tall and sing until he wears out his vocal cords. It is a concert, for crying out loud. A thirty-dollar concert. We should be stoking their fires,
not extinguishing them. They are sure to face bullies and teachers and
bosses and strangers who will thwart their enthusiasm. But not now.
Not tonight. Tonight, they are going to have themselves a real good
time. They feel alive. Don't stop them now.

Listeria Hysteria

Twenty-Four Weeks

WE ARE ON A GETAWAY WITH FRIENDS WHEN IT GETS AWAY FROM ME.

The four of us (and our pups) travel to New Hampshire every fall for a weekend of hiking, foliage, and drinking by the fire. My hiking and drinking abilities are compromised this year, so I know it won't be exactly like past weekends, but I don't predict it will be different in quite this way.

I allow what I expect will be a small release of gas, but I am wrong.

Luckily, I have the upstairs to myself when literal hell breaks loose. I waddle across the hall to the bathroom and find that my underwear is drenched in shame. Such a thing has never happened in my adult life. I can't even remember it happening when I was a child. Now I'll never forget it.

After stuffing my soiled underwear at the bottom of the garbage can and covering it with a heap of crumpled toilet paper, I put on a brave face, go downstairs, and have breakfast with my husband and friends, pretending I'm not a thirty-two-year-old woman who just shit herself a little bit.

"Coffee?" they ask.

"No, thanks."

When we are alone, I admit the accident to Phil. He is not horrified. He is hysterical. (He'll later craft a song parody to the tune of "Beauty and the Beast" that begins, *It's that age-old tale. She thought it was gas. But what came out her ass had substantial mass. Alena shit her pants.*) In the moment, he just says, "Please tell me you were bent over."

happened to you?" I ask.

ensnared by laughter, he smacks his leg. "No," he says, the word into multiple syllables. Then he straightens, and re seriously, "Although I've come close."

his podcast, Dax Shepard admits it happens to him about once ar, a shocking rate of occurrence. His theory is that men are more ggressive in that department, and when you approach flatulence like an extreme sport, you make mistakes. Now it had happened to me. The question was, after thirty years of control, why now?

It had to be listeria.

From the moment the double line sharpens on that pee stick, pamphlets detailing unsafe foods are all but shoved under the bathroom door. Among common no-nos are soft cheeses and deli meat. Why? Listeria, a fanged pathogenic bacterium. If infected, mothers can present with mild fever, headache, and diarrhea—pretty generic symptoms—or they may show no signs at all. You might never realize you are sick while the bacteria seep through your placenta and into your amniotic sac. Infection is extremely dangerous to the baby and can cause miscarriage, premature birth, or stillbirth. The fetal fatality rate is 20 to 30 percent, and the only means of diagnosis is a blood or amniotic fluid culture, a practice no one does regularly.

It's basically every knocked-up woman's nightmare, our version of the boogeyman. Because our immune systems are repressed so as not to reject the fetus, pregnant woman are twenty times more susceptible to being infected with listeria, and because the stakes are so much higher if we become ill, we are read the Tale of Listeriosis at doctors' offices, in books, on chat rooms, and around campfires. Still, listeriosis is pretty rare, even among the expecting. Only twelve in one hundred thousand pregnant women are infected. Might this statistic be higher if we feasted on day-old Subway sandwiches and cold hot dogs like drunken undergraduates? Maybe. But we anticipate the disease as if it's just waiting to pounce on our developing progeny (also like drunken undergraduates).

To defend the buns in our ovens, we shrink away from Italian subs

and farm stands, but the truth is that listeria can exist on virtual[ly]
any food. While there have been more incidences on cold prepared
meats and unpasteurized cheeses, the bacteria have also been found
on chicken, pork, seafood, and vegetables. It's impossible to avoid risk
completely.

Unfortunately, when I get sick, convinced I've been bitten by listeria's venom, I can't defend myself by pointing to the ubiquitous nature
of the bacteria, because I fell prey to the main culprit. I'd stopped for
cider donuts and, overcome by basic white girl autumnal excitement,
lost all sense of pregnancy etiquette. I heaped my arms full of produce, pie, artisanal bread, and a spinach cheese spread made from,
not just any cheese, but feta, a soft cheese, purchased not at a grocery
store chain, where every product is stamped with a pasteurized sticker,
where you couldn't hunt down an unsafe cheese to endanger your life,
but at a farm stand. I am suddenly convinced that, swept up in a whirl-
wind of country wholesomeness, I killed my baby. Death by crudité.

For the next week, I never venture far from a toilet, and whenever
I'm not hovered over that hallowed hollowed seat, by God, I clench
my tush.

I wait four days to call my doctor—I don't want to be that patient
who drops by every time she shits her pants. The call nurse isn't concerned because I don't have a fever, contractions, or bleeding. At twenty-four weeks, the fetus has a 50 percent chance of survival outside the
womb. If I've created a poisonous environment and he's dying inside
me, I think we should free him to offer the kid a fighting chance, so I
ask, "Isn't it worth popping in for an ultrasound?"

"No, it isn't," she says, because I am probably the thirtieth panicked irritated bowel to call that day. (Remember, TGID, Thank God
it's diarrhea.)

Waiting to be struck down by illness, I see symptoms in everything. I wake up sweating and am convinced the fever my thermometer couldn't detect is now breaking. When the fetus goes placid in my
belly, I don't consider that he is small and has repositioned in a way
that makes him more discreet; I am sure my placenta deteriorated and

suffocating. No matter what the nurse says, no matter
 ..band says, no matter what my mother or the Internet
 ..it. My womb is turning into a tomb.

 ..ioia can be funny in retrospect, but at the time, I'm not laugh-
 ..im preparing to grieve. I prearrange what I'll do about the pain-
 ..y futile existence of the furnished nursery. (I knew buying the crib,
 ..hanging table, and car seat so far in advance was premature, but it
was Prime Day! When the boxes were delivered one after the other,
my neighbor asked, "Who is delivering your baby? FedEx or UPS?")
If something happens to the baby now, five and a half months along,
I'll ask a friend to peel off the birch tree decals Phil painstakingly
stuck to the wall, disassemble the furniture, box the clothes and accessories, and pack it all in the attic. I'll call my parents, make sure they
aren't driving, break the news, and let them call other family members.
I'll text everyone else. I won't be able to say it over and over again.
I'll email my students. They might not always pay attention, but even
they'll notice a shrinking stomach.

My gastrointestinal issues clear after a week. A day or so later, the
baby shifts and I again feel his movements. I palm my stomach, wait
for his touch, and we hold hands through the universe that separates
us. I am comforted by these developments, but I sense that confidence is tenuous, and will remain only until the next bout of irregularity. When I deliver the baby, my focus will shift, and I'll zero in on
his abnormalities. I'll count the ounces he drank or didn't. I'll tune in
to every rash. I'll analyze every off-color poo. I'll live in the agony
between his breaths.

This must be what it means to cradle something I don't want to
lose, to care, maybe even to love—a constant hum of anxiety in my
ears, a worried preoccupation, an endless series of listeria hysterias
until my poor restless heart wears out.

Letter to Baby

Twenty-Seven Weeks

Dear Baby,

It's six thirty on a November morning. The branches outside the window are almost bare. My belly is hard and globed, like half the world is hanging off my middle.

The sparrows are beginning to wake, and so are you, Baby. You're rolling around my stomach, stretching, yawning, maybe. Are you a morning person like your dad? Will the two of you tiptoe in the tranquil hours while I sleep in? Or is time warped in your dark, humid incubator, and when you emerge into the exacting sunshine of this world, will you be cranky and scowl against the light of morning, like me, your mama?

We're almost through the second trimester, you and me. You're as big as a cabbage. Your eyes are beginning to open. You've grown hair. You can hear my voice.

Hello, Baby.

We've reached an important milestone. If you came now (don't come now), you'd likely be okay. You are no longer absolutely dependent on my body. You'd have a rough start, but you could do it. You'd survive on your own. Don't take that as a hint. You can stay where you are. You still need to practice breathing and gain weight. So get comfortable. One of us should.

We've called you several things since we learned of you. Lately we are trying out Rowen.

Rowan is what the Irish call a red-berried mountain ash, a tree whose roots sink deep to thrive amidst the inhospitable soil of a rocky hillside. (Read between

nhospitable soil.) If we go with that name, we'll swap the a for
u ours. Even with a name, we have no idea who you'll become.

extent, you will be a shifting viscous thing that will never stop trans-
you sample different characteristics, as various factors in your environ-
fluence you, and as your priorities and personhood evolve. But maybe the
of you will remain steady. I know I can't be predestining, but I do have a
sh list. Here it is. No pressure.

I hope you'll be goofy—not too proud or self-conscious to embrace silliness
wholeheartedly. I hope you'll be curious, that you'll find the world a fascinating
place with mysteries compelling you to turn every rock and check behind every door.
I hope you'll smile and laugh easily. I hope you'll, for the most part, be unendingly
kind—unless the person in question is not deserving of your kindness. I hope
you'll have that rare quality that makes others feel special, the way your great
grandfather does. I hope you won't feel superior to those around you, and if good
fortune gives you a leg up, that you'll offer your hand to pull your neighbor to your
height. I hope you'll be compulsively honest, willing to share secrets that verge on the
embarrassing, because this promotes intimacy, humility, and human connection. I
hope you'll be optimistic. There is plenty of darkness in this world, so it doesn't
take much effort to stay in the shadows; the lucky ones gravitate toward the light,
and the ones who aren't so lucky, but who are smart, work their way there. I hope
you'll realize there is always more to learn, always room for self-improvement, and
yet be wise enough to love and forgive yourself for your imperfections, because we're
all crazy and flawed in a million different ways.

Some of these traits you'd inherit from me, but most are the reasons I fell in
love with your father. He may be silly and gracious and a more conscientious cook,
but I'm wittier and more intuitive and have a party trick memory for personal
details, which comes in handy more often than you'd think. He seems like the
easy choice for favorite parent, but sometimes he forgets to check the toilet to see if
everything flushed down, so don't be so quick to decide.

I don't know what kind of a person you'll turn into and in what ways you'll
change. I look forward to meeting all of your versions.

For now, all we know is that you're ours, and maybe that's enough. I felt
this acutely when the hospital explained that they are going to give the three of
us—and only us—matching bracelets. Mom, Dad, and Baby. Distinct family

markers. It's for security purposes, but it feels a lot like belonging.

Your father and I have been a team of two for almost a decade now (plus Penny—you've already heard her bark at the cat across the street. Your dad says the only way you can disappoint him is if you don't love her. It sounds like a joke, but he's serious). You'll become the third human member of our team. Welcome.

I don't know what kind of mother I'll be. This is what I mean when I say our identities continue to evolve. When you arrive, I'll be meeting a new part of myself, and a new aspect of your father—a completely altered team dynamic.

You aren't even out yet and I already fear I'm a bad mother. I've slept on my back, which can cut off your blood flow. I've even slept on my stomach—but I suppose telling you that is like breaking that news to a bug you just squished. I've sipped glasses of wine and nibbled cold pepperoni.

Worst of all, I'm not experiencing the sentiment, the connection, that so many expectant mothers gush over. These women post photos of their ever-growing belly alongside the fruit or vegetable that captures the size of their fetus, with captions like "My love grows right alongside you." Maybe I shouldn't be telling you this, Baby, but I'm not sure I love you yet. Not exactly. I'd be devastated if I lost you, because that would mean losing your possibilities and the future I've imagined, but can you really love somebody you've never met? I look forward to meeting you, getting to know you, and getting to know the part of me that is your mother. I look forward to loving you. But I'm not sure I love you yet, and in the deepest part of me, the darkest part I can't bear to look at for long, I am terrified our bond will never form. I sense the deficit of love, or at least a certain type of love, persisting like a storm cloud.

Maybe this is why, at the end of prenatal workout videos, when the instructor encourages me to cradle my belly and connect with the life and love growing inside me, to breathe around the baby and picture each breath as a hug, I turn the video off. I consider the workout done. I can't bring myself to connect, not honestly, not in that honeyed way. But maybe what I'm feeling is normal, and the love will rush in as you slide out.

We're going to try hard to do right by you, but I'm sure we'll make mistakes. We'll snap over something small because it feels large in the moment. We'll get lazy and stop paying attention just long enough for you to tumble from the couch or make your way through the cabinet beneath the kitchen sink. We won't teach you the best way you know how to learn. We'll want our own space. We may even sometimes miss when we were just a two-person team. Maybe we'll accidentally instill guilt or shame in you. It happens all the time.

One day you'll look at us and see our flaws for the first time. After years of believing I always have the answers, that I'm beautiful and kind and dependable, you'll realize I'm controlling and selfish and starting to get old lady neck, that sometimes I say things even though I know it'll make someone feel bad. You'll mistake your dad's introversion for apathy. His stiffness will appear more awkward than contemplative, and his beloved wool will begin to smell musty. You'll have to come to grips with the truth that your parents are human, just as we learned, and are continually reminded, that our own parents are human. This new reality may be a struggle to reconcile. It may be disappointing. Heartbreaking, even. Forgive us.

Just as I'll forgive you when you grow up despite my best efforts. When you say you hate me, your mother, the woman who hauled you around in her womb for the longest forty weeks of her life, whose body continues to carry the cells you left behind. When you lie. When you endanger your life, the most precious thing to me. When you want your own space. When you send my calls to voicemail. When you don't come home for the holidays. When you inevitably leave me for someone else, someone you—rightly—love better, and begin your own team.

I'm looking into the future now, so far down the passageway of your life it's tapering into a point. There is much between now and then: sleepless nights, breastfeeding, diapers, cradle cap, and fevers. And even before that: contractions, pushing, crowning.

As I lie in bed with your dad and dog—with you—I shudder at the price I will have to pay to meet you, but I'm confident you'll be worth every groan, every drop of blood.

Still, when you're ready to come out and unveil who you are to me, your dad, and the rest of the world, try to suck it in, won't you? We have a long relationship ahead, and you can't underestimate the value of first impressions.

Love,

Your Mama

PART IV

Third Trimester

Second Letter to My Body

Twenty-Eight Weeks

Dear Body,

Remember when I wanted to develop that definitively pregnant but adorable belly that moms-to-be flaunt on social media?

I was so young then.

That preggo bump is apparently only cute on skinny women who remain skinny everywhere else, the waifs who look like they swallowed a soccer ball. That isn't me. I look like I've swallowed a soccer banquet. I've never been skinny. At some points I've been solid, sturdy, maybe even lean, but never skinny. Now my thick arms and legs are matched by my protruding gut. Against all reason, I have Dad Bod.

With twelve weeks to go, I've already put on twenty-one pounds. It's not looking like I'll steady at twenty-five, the lower end of the recommended weight gain. I'll be lucky if I'm inside the upper limit of thirty-five. Worse still, now it's winter, and when I go to the doctor's office, I'm not wearing cotton shorts and a tank top. The scale has to contend with the bulk of denim, sweaters, and boots. Would it be too vain to shimmy into a sundress before my next appointment and sit in the waiting room dressed for a cookout beside the other patients in their scarves and peacoats?

Before I got pregnant, I restricted my dessert intake to two a week. Now that

I'm heavy with child and finally nausea-free (praise Aphrodite, goddess of fertility), I feel the discomforts and sacrifices of my life entitle me to a cookie or six. Desserts are back on the table, which I've extended by inserting all the leaves. This might have something to do with my weight gain. Or it might be the four servings of Cheez-Its I stuff into my face to absorb the stomach acid that shoots up my esophagus.

Maybe I should embrace this period, the first and only time it's socially acceptable to bound into a room belly first, when people shouldn't interpret my weight gain as defeat, but rather a mark of accomplishment, a sign of all that I am creating. But just because people shouldn't judge doesn't mean they don't. Being pregnant is a bit of a performance—the excitement I affected in my announcements, pretending not to be so sick, emphasizing my not drinking—and there are the Muppet hecklers on the balcony, jeering every unnecessary pound and slovenly outfit.

Then there's the rubber popper toy of my belly button, which is beginning the process of flipping inside out. Maybe it's like those temperature gauges on turkeys; when the button pops into a full outie, dinner is done.

It isn't just my stomach. There's cellulose where there's never been cellulose before, like the inside of my biceps—fat is beginning to curdle beneath my skin. My nose is broadening. My nose. My neck is absorbing everything around it. My jaw needs a search and rescue team to pull it out of its sinkhole before it's too late. This (or my turkey thermometer belly button) inspired a dream last night, in which I looked in the mirror and saw a wattle hanging from my jowls.

My body has never changed so quickly, so completely. It's getting so that I don't recognize myself. I was getting old before, no longer that twenty-year-old in a tiny bikini so everyone can enjoy my perky form and elastic skin. You're welcome, world! (My mournful brain has airbrushed history so that I was basically a Sports Illustrated model.) Pregnancy has accelerated the aging process. It's like the baby is sucking out my life force, stealing my youth like Bette Midler in Hocus Pocus.

My abdominals have been front-kicked apart by a tiny action hero in slow motion. My tired boobs plunk atop my belly like an orangutan's. Lines remain around my mouth even when I stop smiling (like after seeing my reflection, for instance). And my muscles spasm when I reach for toilet paper that is adhered too far back on the wall.

Body, you've left the station, and you've got a one-way ticket going downhill. I suppose I may as well throw my cottage cheese arms up and enjoy the ride.

Your begrudging passenger,

Me

What to Doula

Twenty-Nine Weeks

WHEN I CONFESS DELIVERY ANXIETY TO MY OBSTETRICIAN (HONESTLY, I'M shaking in my hospital booties), she says the degree of my worry is a concern itself, and something of an odity. According to her, most women aren't terrified, which seems as inappropriate a response as it must be inaccurate. What's not to dread? Active labor lasts an average of twelve hours for first-time mothers. I don't even like 5Ks. I'm not looking forward to Lucifer's Ironman when my training has been nine months of potato chips and couch cushions.

I might pass out from labor pain. I might push so hard I shit on the table. They might have to sever the place between my vagina and asshole. Although Phil will be there, I'm afraid I'll feel quite alone, and will resent him for not being able to help me. I'm afraid, when the nurse leaves the room and it's just us, we won't know what to do.

And I take issue that this doctor can so easily stand across from a patient, shuddering over the journey she must travel, and dismiss the epic feat of motherhood, tell her she's wrong to feel daunted, and alone in her wrongness. Doctor Tough Girl goes on to warn that my anxiety could make labor more difficult, since tensed-up muscles would prevent the baby from dropping. This, needless to say, doesn't help my anxiety.

Who does help is my friend Amy, who swears she felt more confident after hiring a doula.

Doula is an ancient Greek word for "woman's servant," but since that phrase only seems appropriate if discussing *Downton Abbey*, let's call her a nonmedical birth coach. She explores your hopes for the experience (simple—I hope I survive it): hospital or birth center, epidural or alternative pain management (I'll take the heartiest epidural on the menu, please!), music or silence, touch or solitary, light or dark, bed or tub. (I love me a bath, but stewing in my own blood while someone uses a pool skimmer to extract my poop sounds like a scene from *Saw*.) She educates about the progression of events and possible outcomes.

She meets you at your home or the hospital when labor begins and doesn't leave you until two hours post-delivery. She repositions you every twenty minutes, comforts, guides your breathing, massages, and applies counterpressure to ease your pain. She administers aromatherapy. She assists you into a warm tub to loosen your muscles, encourage the baby to drop, and reduce the severity of vaginal tearing. (Reduce, not eliminate. She isn't magic; you're probably going to tear, girl.) During the pushing phase, she assesses your physical state, recommends positions, mentors, and holds your leg so your husband doesn't get an orchestra seat to your Little Shop of Horrors. After delivery, she helps with breastfeeding and visits the following day and two weeks later to check for postpartum red flags. Doulas are fairy godmothers there to transform a sweating, dilating, bleeding, mucous secreting young maiden into a mother—although it's never as easy as bibbidi-bobbidi-boo.

My friend found her doula through our shared OB-GYN, who recommends only one. Like many female superstars—Oprah, Beyoncé, Madonna—this doula is referred to by first name alone.

Enza is a hardy five-foot-nothing Italian American with a low center of gravity, silver hair that falls in waves to her shoulders, and a youthful face capable of capturing somberness and joy in equal measure. In our preliminary meeting, she doesn't sugarcoat labor, explaining it calmly and confidently. When Phil and I joke about my vomiting style, she breaks into full-bodied laughter.

She's both passionate and compassionate, saying, "If you think

I could help you but you can't afford my fee, we can come to some other agreement. I do this because I love it."

As a person with financial hesitations (I'm cheap), I'm tempted to negotiate. Phil, though, reminds me that we are privileged to be able to afford it, and Enza should save her discounts for those truly in need. This is the price of marrying a good person.

Having assisted in over 250 deliveries, Enza has seen some shit, figuratively and literally. While this will be Phil's and my first time, she's seasoned. She'll know when things are abnormal. She can reassure and offer wisdom, or a second opinion if I worry that the doctor is rushing into unnecessary procedures. Her methods of pain relief might delay me from asking for (demanding) an epidural, which can slow labor and increase the need for emergency surgery.

Enza is our comfort, and our insurance. I'd rather have help that wasn't required than feel lost or overwhelmed and wish she were there. After our first meeting, some anxiety evaporates. I feel less alone.

My parents, DIYers and the most fiscally efficient people I've ever met, aren't so convinced. They are the people who fill their cars up across town because that station is two cents cheaper, embarking in a caravan with extra travel tanks if they have gas rewards. They dry and reuse paper towels and Ziploc bags. Instead of buying vegetable stock, my mom pours water from steamed vegetables into a Tupperware she stores in the freezer; if I forget and dump broccoli water down the sink, she gasps. In forty years, they've never paid for garbage pickup, hauling it to the dump themselves, or worse, scurrying around the Shaw's dumpster in the dark like a couple of middle-aged raccoons.

When they ask what I get for my doula investment, I cobble together an answer about pain relief. My mother says, "That's what an epidural is for," and my father adds, "I've had twenty-seven surgeries and never hired a doula." One of his female friends made the mistake of telling him that kidney stones are the pain equivalent of childbirth, and he's gripped onto that like a certificate of achievement.

This judgment is a common pulse beneath the subject of maternal care, particularly when it comes to methods of pain relief, as if the more suffering a woman can endure, the more credit she earns. Never mind the ten months leading up to the big day. (Forty weeks of pregnancy falls between nine and ten months. Some countries, like South Korea, round up, but perhaps not surprisingly, Americans round down. Not me!) After the odyssey of pregnancy, we expect women to grin and bear the climax because we have this sick way of prizing female pain, especially in childbirth, the most female of acts. If you don't feel the heat of every contraction, the sear of every push, you surrendered and don't get to iron that badge on your sash.

When women describe their birth experience, they often feel the need to acknowledge their concessions, like "I tried for as long as I could, but I was so worn out; I had to get an epidural," as if this is a defeat rather than the shrewd use of a practical resource.

There's similar reproach when recruiting a doula. If a man outsources, we call it delegating, but women who leverage extra support are considered indulgent, weak, or too incompetent to accomplish the task on their own.

The World Health Organization recommends doulas for all, because birth companions can recognize emergencies and alert healthcare workers, who are often absent during labor. This is no small matter, considering half of maternal fatalities in delivery could be prevented through timely intervention, and the maternal death rate in the United States is the highest in the developing world. It has increased by 26 percent in recent years, now hovering around 23 in 100,000, which is double the rate of listeriosis in pregnancy, and yet women are rarely versed in the benefits of a doula, while always lectured on unpasteurized cheese, which suggests the ways in which we protect the fetus versus the mother.

Doulas can literally be a matter of life or death, and shouldn't just be esteemed, but covered by insurance. But why does it have to be life or death for women's issues to be taken seriously? Why can't a woman's *quality* of life be enough?

Instead of using pain tolerance to appraise a mother's performance, we should scrap the assessment altogether and instead—I don't know—make her comfortable and happy. She is performing an act of service to humanity. Creating life is hard enough without pressuring women to make it as hard as possible in order to garner respect.

I may be in my thirties and about to become a mother in my own right, but I sometimes still have to remind myself that I don't need my parents to sign my permission slip. In this case, I'm bolstering my bench with as many support people and experts as possible. It's my delivery, my body, my choice, and since Oprah isn't available, I choose Enza.

Ache You Tailfeather

Thirty Weeks

OTHER WOMEN IN THIS STAGE OF PREGNANCY LOOK POSITIVELY DIVINE, like Mother Earth herself, each strand of hair a velvety rope, embers smoldering beneath her skin, hands posed on the orb of her creation, eyes cast serenely toward the future. I look more like a toad. *Ribbit, ribbit.* Or, when it comes to my inseams, *Rip it, rip it.*

I know I'm looking bedraggled because people have begun to ask, "Are you starting to feel uncomfortable?" If by uncomfortable, they mean debilitating pain as my organs, bones, and joints are rearranged and bashed like this kid is break-dancing in my abdomen, then yeah, I'm starting to feel uncomfortable.

Pain pulses in my back, neck, and pelvis. I lose my breath walking up my stairs, and I live in a split-level. That's five steps. While Phil wraps my late-grandmother's wool shawl around his shoulders, I've stripped down to a T-shirt and shorts and still there's steam rising off my clammy skin. Heartburn lures me from sleep with an acidic tendril curling from my belly to my throat. My skin is dry. I've lost circulation in one arm. The baby's head presses against sacral nerves and triggers a bolt of crotch lightning so shocking it takes my breath away.

The non-pregnant employ euphemisms like "uncomfortable" to make themselves more comfortable. To look plainly at the pain women tolerate, the double standards they overcome, the many responsibilities and multifaceted identities they juggle, would be to look directly into the sun.

I've been spared many pregnancy discomforts: hemorrhoids, hyperthyroidism, UTIs, insomnia, dragon-breath heartburn (not to get too technical), and perhaps worst of all, hyperemesis gravidarum. It sounds like a Harry Potter unforgiveable curse because it is. God bless these women who suffer sickness so severe they are dehydrated and hospitalized, nine tortuous months that feel like death and often end up that way, risking their lives for the sake of another, a condition so emotionally, mentally, and physically eviscerating, it often results in PTSD. To manage symptoms, women do everything to dull their senses, avoiding television, toothpaste, car rides, and showers—showers—because the sensation of too much water hitting their skin could make them puke. Basically, until her baby is born, a pregnant woman with HG has to hole up in her house alone, unbathed, without stimulation. Yet, some choose to do pregnancy all over again. This is courage I'll never know.

I also don't have to contend with obstacles faced by women of color: most troublingly, a mortality rate three times that of white women, 60 percent of which might have been prevented if transportation, healthcare coverage, or work schedules hadn't precluded medical appointments, or if their distress were taken more seriously during office visits.

I push myself up from the couch (because that's how I get up from anything these days—by sort of thrusting off of it) and pain scorches the center of my ass, so deep I can't touch it. If I was a drug mule, I hurt at the heroin packets. I'm not familiar enough with anatomy to articulate what exactly is hurting, so I demonstrate as best I can. Wearing only a shirt and underwear, I turn away from Phil, bend over, and dig my fingers into my butt crack.

"It hurts here, in the bone. What is this?" I ask.

"I don't know what you're pointing to. Your fingers disappeared a couple inches ago."

I text my friend Andrea, the physician assistant, a word visual of the issue. The answer bounces back immediately: my tailbone.

Tailbone pain is common in the third trimester. Your body, namely your ovaries, placenta, and uterus, have been releasing the hormone relaxin, which sounds like a beach vacation, and it is, but only if, on the last day of that beach vacation, you suffer a zip-lining accident and are shipped home in a full body cast.

The hormone is responsible for a lot of good in childbearing and birthing: it promotes implantation, prevents early contractions, stimulates blood flow to the placenta, and relaxes the cervix, vagina, and pelvic ligaments to ease delivery. But universal ligament and joint relaxation isn't without consequences. Wobbly joints don't bear weight as well, and pregnancy involves extra weight—in my case, a lot of it. Relaxin is the reason my friend knew she was pregnant even when the test read negative. She experienced pain reminiscent of her previous pregnancy, when vertebrae in her lower back loosened, deteriorating necessary support in her spine, and she had to scoot down the stairs on her bum.

Relaxin is the bugger behind my tailbone pain. The hormone stretches the pelvic floor, which shifts the coccyx. Then there's the little bodybuilder in my belly, bulking up on protein shakes, doing squats atop my slackened joints and nerves.

I follow the recommendations for relief I turn up on the Internet: stretches and belly taping. It ironically doesn't seem possible to achieve child's pose with my obtrusive belly, but I slowly, carefully, arch and curve my spine in a cow-cat stretch, and then clumsily flop over and drive my crotch toward the ceiling into a bridge. Since I can't see or access the underside of my mounded middle, Phil tapes my gut, affording my bump a happy pumpkin face I can view only in the mirror.

The piercing subsides to a pang overnight. Finally, something worked! The sudden absence of pain is thrilling, a pleasure itself. I'd feared this soreness was just a new part of me until the baby arrived, making for an unbearable ten weeks. Now it's been banished with a few simple tricks. Thank you, tape—you sweet, sweet, miracle, reinforcing my belly to my hips. My gratitude is euphoric.

• • • • •

My skin begins to sting twelve hours later. One edge of the tape has come unstuck; I figure it got yanked, and that's what tingled my skin. But it's fine. What's a little irritation compared to all the good the tape is doing?

It's angrier the next morning. I try to ignore it, to forgive the tape its flaws, but by that night, Phil notices the effects. "Maybe you should take the tape off," he says.

"The directions said I could leave it on for three days," I insist, protesting too much.

"Are you *afraid* to take it off?"

"No." To prove him wrong, I tug on the undone edge. My skin shrieks and I whimper. Now the exposed skin isn't just red. It's rippling.

"Maybe you should try removing it in a hot shower."

Hot water pelts me and I pray it soaks through the adhesive. After a few minutes, I pluck at the loose edge. The tape clings. Is it possible the water made it stickier? It doesn't matter—the tape has to go. This shower is a showdown. A tape-à-tête.

I grit my teeth and peel. It feels so caustic, I half expect to look down and find Rowen waving to me through a little tape-shaped window.

Phil hears me moan and yells, "Wait! Maybe it's oil based."

I don't know what that means, but it includes waiting, so I listen.

Moments later, he whips the shower curtain aside, brandishing a canister of cooking spray in one hand, and reveals me, naked, ballooned, dripping with water, and sniveling, blue tape dangling from my distended middle, a trail of bubbled skin in its wake. He digs deep to resist my sex appeal, cranks off the water, and dabs my belly with a towel. Then he uncaps his culinary elixir and spews oil onto my belly like I'm a human baking sheet. When it trickles onto the exposed raw skin, I feel like I am being broiled.

I massage the lubricant into the cotton strip. (What a waste of the words "massage" and "lubricant.") The oil shaves the teeth off the adhesive. I pull millimeter by careful millimeter, anticipating sting all the way. Soon I see what is so painful: the tape inflamed my skin into blisters, which the tape then uncapped.

As I towel off, I catch a glimpse of my stomach in the bathroom mirror. The scalded wound transformed my happy pumpkin into a gruesome jack-o'-lantern.

Phil applies ointment and gauze. I cradle my sack of baby and go pitifully to sleep.

• • • • •

My tailbone remains quiet, but the spotlight shifts to my pelvic floor, who, apparently, has just been waiting for her chance to croon. With every step, she sings as if I underwent an aggressive gynecological exam, or as if the fetus is trying to dig its way out. Sometimes I look down expecting to find a tiny Tim, from *Shawshank Redemption*, not *A Christmas Carol*.

My groin ligaments feel like two rubber bands pulled taut, like an unimaginative middle schooler was charged with crafting a harness to support my baby (no offense, God). My doctor cheerfully says there is no treatment, definitely no cure, except delivery, of course.

I spring for a U-shape pregnancy pillow, a monstrosity that loops behind my head and down both sides of my body, eating up half our king bed. I tumble inside and am unaware of heartbeats beyond my downy cloud. If Phil wants my attention, he has to yell from the bottom like Prince Charming to Rapunzel, except I don't let down my hair.

I stretch. I Kegel all over town: in my living room, my car, as I type this sentence, unbeknownst to my fellow library patrons. I do prenatal yoga. I strap myself into front-paneled maternity pants. I finally get a prenatal massage. I shimmy into a bellyband. I soak in a tub. (Not too warm or I'm a bad mama. Not too cold or I'll get pneumonia and kill my baby, like a bad mama.) I use muscle-relaxing bath salts. I ice my parts and apply heat. I try walking, and then I don't walk. I sit on a lumbar pillow, and then a non-lumbar pillow. Nothing works.

As I'm nursing my crotchety crotch, my lower back freezes. Relaxin turned my joints and ligaments to taffy, so my muscles responded, *Join together, ladies. It's up to us to hold this bag of bones together.*

Before, when I saw a pregnant woman waddling, I assumed it was a balance issue. Now I know the truth—she is in pain. (Or, maybe, she shit herself.) Perhaps this is just what the third trimester looks like. Still, I can't bring myself to surrender to agony with so many more weeks to endure. Not yet.

I ditch the bellyband, which I suspect is responsible for the back tightness, and consider the tape again, but the wound from my first attempt has already left a scar. How many more marks will this baby leave behind?

Love at First Touch

Thirty-One Weeks

MY PRENATAL MASSEUSE PERFORMS THE LORD'S WORK. ON HER TABLE, I'M not just a baby-making machine, a vessel with a singular purpose, but a person in my own right. I feel human again, experiencing pleasure rather than niggles and stabs. Sometimes I don't even realize how tight my back muscles are until her fingers carve out pebbles I've secretly stored in my shoulders and along my spine, releasing tension and a flood of endorphins. I've had massages before, but not like this. She plays my knots like piano keys and my constricted cells open and rejoice, becoming part of her symphony. I hear the hallelujah choir of angels singing me to sleep. If this is love, and I think it might be, maybe I've never truly loved anyone before.

If I were to assign her number a photo in my cell phone, it'd be a stream of light slicing through cumulus clouds. If she moved, I'd consider relocating to be near her. I might name this woman godmother to our unborn child. I might add her as a beneficiary to my husband's life insurance policy. If she's accused of a crime, I'll be her alibi. If she's put behind bars despite my efforts, I'll divorce Phil and marry her for the conjugal visits in which she'll rub my back and I'll pay her in tender kisses and commissary funds.

Her massages could end family disputes. Government shutdowns. They could be massages for peace.

She is, no surprise, rated the best massage therapist on the North Shore of Boston. I happened to discover her business on a day she had a rare cancellation. If that's not fate, fate doesn't exist.

After our initial meeting, I was heartbroken to hear she didn't have another opening for six weeks. How could I survive without her—without ever feeling *good*? My life and body were transforming (degrading) so quickly; I had no idea what I'd be doing, how I'd be feeling, what I'd look like, who I'd become, six weeks from that first massage. But I was sure of one thing—I'd be curled up on her table, inside the pillow nest my mama robin builds when she knows I'm coming.

Appointments with her are the only items on otherwise blank calendar pages, and they are penned in thick, permanent marker. In between visits, I live small, stiff lifetimes. If I had a massage scheduled the day of a friend's funeral, I'd have to really think about how much that friend meant to me. (Did they ever offer me a massage?)

Once in a while, I slip in a last-minute appointment because someone else cancelled, and I wonder what tragedy must have struck to make that person sacrifice precious time on the altar of muscular relief. Did she go into active labor? Witness a mob hit and is on the lamb? Did she get into a horrific car crash? A minor collision would not do; I'd still limp my scraped-up ass across town. For a heartbeat, I feel sorry for that person and the gratification they lost, likely not to be experienced again until the weather has changed. I grieve in reverential solidarity as I click the button to book her spot.

If there was a killing spree in our area, I wouldn't be surprised to hear the victims all had upcoming massage appointments. Not that I'm saying I'd murder anyone myself—I'm not crazy, although pain can drive a person to do crazy things—but maybe another client is a closeted psychopath, willing to do the unthinkable just to clear the calendar of a local massage genius. Even psychopaths need sixty minutes of tender loving care.

On the First Day of Christmas, Do Not Say to Me

Thirty-Two Weeks

1. (On the phone to someone else): Yes, she looks *very* pregnant.

2. Do you need to sit down? You look like you need to sit down.

3. Look at that plate. Eating for two!

4. Oh, careful. There's whiskey in that cake. (Give me a slice before I eat you.)

5. Will someone bring the car around? For God's sake, look at her.

6. Does anyone want wine? Or Alena, soda?

7. That coffee better be decaf. I don't care what they say.

8. You're all belly. (And brains and a fat ass too.)

9. Do you have bigger shirts for next month? That one looks like it's stretched as far as it can go.

10. When a woman has a boy she carries all in front. When she has a girl she's wide all around. I thought you were having a girl.

Farewell to Breasts

Thirty-Three Weeks

As an adolescent, I knelt before the mirror in half-filled A cups, praying I wouldn't inherit the Irish chest of my father's family. I was chubby. The perk of being chubby was supposed to be ample boobs, and yet my torso could have been mistaken for that of a little video gamer, or the boy at the pool who bounces on the edge of a diving board, jiggling from knee to chin. In fact, one of my middle school friends informed me that I had fat kid nipples. I didn't know what she meant at the time, but it turns out she was making a medically significant observation, albeit without any bedside manner. Later, my doctor would be genteel enough to call them flat, not fat.

By the time I turned eighteen, I'd welcomed hearty Sicilian breasts with the jubilant relief of the prodigal son's father. (I suspect he was a boob man.) Like everything, they came with their own consequences. I had to exercise with straitjacket sports bras, and backless dresses were the stuff of legend, but those breasts became symbols of my femininity and sexuality. (Sadly, I'd go on to marry an ass man. What a waste.)

Now they are being slowly stripped of that sensuality. My nipples have darkened, expanded, and speckled, and are either flaking dry skin or producing colostrum crusts. They bloat on my inflated rib cage like two loaves of dough. They've swollen from D to DD so quickly, the friction has produced skin tags, what WebMD defines as "a small flap of tissue that hangs off the skin by a connecting stalk." That description puts the bone in bona fide old lady moles, and takes it out of everything else.

As if skin stalks weren't bad enough, thanks to a lowered immune system, hormones, and my constant state of damp, I've developed a rash between my breasts. The nurse at my doctor's office suspects it's a yeast infection. (Gross!) She was so unimpressed by the prospect, she didn't even ask me to come in; pregnant women have problems more deserving of medical attention than fungal infections. She advised I clean and dry the area, apply antifungal and hydrocortisone cream, and expose my boobs to air.

Where I was once desirable, now I'm topless on my bed, as alluring as a beached elephant seal or, for that matter, as a skin tag. I've traded in what we've been taught is the most prized trait of a woman (her sexuality) for the next stage of value—her procreation. This is a misogynist view, I know, and yet I grieve the loss of the former. I feel I've been drained of my power, without yet appreciating my new capability.

I'm less like a Russian nesting doll and more like a galaxy, stars splitting and rearranging to form constellations, moons orbiting, and planets spinning on their axes. Every particle, every speck of dust, is its own miracle contributing to the seemingly infinite firmament. Who knows what my baby will go on to do, the lives he'll affect or create? I contain a solar system, and if God is the creator of the universe, then God is She. Make way for the Milky Way.

But there is still the sad state of my breasts: bumpy, red, and drooped in defeat, as if they know their glory days are behind them. Yet, there is so much ahead. They are about to make their most important contributions, sustaining life, churning up enough nourishment to feed another person. That's hard, essential, and noble work—more than enough to make anyone look a little rundown. They're demonstrating a hell of a lot more skill than any male breast, and yet they still have to worry about how they look, what they're wearing, and their bad attitude.

Isn't that just typical?

In My Condition

Thirty-Four Weeks

MY OBSTETRICIAN GLIDES THE WAND OF THE FETAL HEART RATE MONITOR over my belly, and from beneath the machine's static rises that familiar gushing rhythm. This time, though, the tempo is accompanied by another beat, a sporadic snare against the steady bass drum.

"He's hiccupping," the doctor says.

Ultrasounds are small but precious glimpses that make tangible the concept of the resident inside my biosphere, but this vocalization is a particularly customized message from another world, near to me but so apart: My *son* has the *hiccups*. He's a boy who hit the amniotic fluid too hard. A single leaf of fondness stirs around my heart.

I want to know more about him, to see him beyond the pulse of heart, lungs, and hiccups, but I really don't want to do what I have to do to make that happen.

I don't know when, I don't know for how long, but there will be a degree and brand of pain I've never experienced before (and, like the Daniel Day-Lewis film, there will also be blood). There is a baby in my belly, and he can't stay there. My pain is his only way out.

How do I go about my daily tasks—brewing coffee, grocery shopping, waving to my neighbor—knowing trauma is imminent? It's like telling someone, "Go on. Walk around the block. You may or may not be beaten by a baseball bat this time, but you *definitely* will be beaten by a baseball bat eventually."

I just pray labor doesn't strike in the middle of a nor'easter, because I'm not delivering at home. I don't care what it takes to get within arm's reach of medical experts and an epidural, even if it means Phil and Penny dragging me on a toboggan.

When the sky grays, I cross my legs.

· · · · ·

I don't consider what ten centimeters of dilation really means until my doula compares it to the size of a New York City bagel. That's how large the opening of my cervix will get. By the transition phase of birth, the obstetrician can flip me upside down and use my vaginal canal as a soup tureen to dish out sustenance to his staff before delivery. This, unfortunately, isn't the most disturbing revelation of Enza's childbirth tutorial.

The pushing phase of delivery lasts an average of three and a half hours for first-time mothers. When she tells me this, I'm sure she has misspoken. Three and half hours is the length of the movie *Titanic*. I can't have a human stuck between my legs for as long as it takes Leonardo DiCaprio to go from a young treat to a frozen one. When depicted on the silver screen, that part of the birth lasts only three *minutes*. Sure, it looks like hell. The actress's neck veins bulge and her face gets red and moist—all of which, oddly, only enhances her beauty—but it's one scene, so the portrayal isn't overly daunting; you can endure almost anything for a scene. But three and a half hours? I hardly have enough stamina to watch *Lord of the Rings*, never mind strain through my own Middle-earth.

Enza agitates a baby doll's head against the heel of her hand, bumping again and again to demonstrate how pushes crest the baby over the pelvic bone. She describes it as rocking a tire out of a ditch. Each push applies gas on and off. I can't concentrate on metaphors. All I can think about are the literal implications: the baby's forehead, and then its nose, scraping my bone. My baby. My bone. Three and a half hours of getting him over the ledge of my pelvis and down through the shoot.

Then Enza describes the ring of fire, a Johnny Cash–style

nightmare. When the baby's head squeezes through my canal, his head will mash against capillaries and nerves, making it feel like my crotch is burning and my asshole is about to explode. While such a sensation might tempt me to tighten my tunnel muscles, to yank the umbilical cord and lasso the baby back into my womb where he isn't singeing my innards with his flaming crown, I'll have to work against my instincts and push, push, push. Probably poop a little too. But if I'm directed to stop pushing, I must hear the order amidst my agony and terror, and obey immediately, because that means the umbilical cord is wrapped around my baby's neck.

These pushes are still weeks away, but I'm getting light-headed just thinking about them. Enza asks if I'm feeling all right, but how can I be, knowing this is my fate any minute? I always considered myself to be tough, especially "for a girl." I practiced martial arts for five years, receiving blows that darkened my eyes and shattered bone. I took boxing classes and prided myself in the mini orchids of blood vessels that flowered between my knuckles. But the prospect of this otherworldly pain spins the phrase "for a girl" on its head. *Tough for a girl* shouldn't qualify the resilience, but amplify it to the highest level.

I'm starting to think I'm not tough, especially not for a girl, and to answer Enza's question, no, I'm not feeling all right.

• • • • •

Friends and family attempt the typical reassurances: women have been going through this for thousands of years, it'll all be worth it, you won't even remember the pain. I don't find these platitudes comforting. People have been dying for thousands of years, but we still fear death, and colonoscopies are worthwhile but we still prefer to keep our rectums to ourselves.

The last encouragement—the "you won't remember the pain" bit—is all well and good for distant-future me. But what about near-future me? She's the one who will be breathing through contractions. She's the one who shouldn't eat foods like granola or Triscuits because their sharp edges will scrape the insides of her throat when she vomits. She's the one whose vaginal canal will have to stretch into a turtleneck around the head of a human. She's the one whose tender skin will tear, whose organs will shift, who will be sweating and crying and moaning like an animal. In the days following delivery, she'll be the one with the finger of a frozen glove shimmied up her hoo-ha while a tiny stranger fusses and poops black tar and gnaws at nipples that were once sexual and are now cracked soft-serve handles. She'll bleed copiously for days in the menstruation version of the *Game of Thrones* Red Wedding. Her pelvic floor will be stretched and floppy for up to a year—maybe forever. What about her? Is her distress discounted because it was necessary for creation, worthwhile in comparison to the value of new life, plenty of other women have done it, and eventually it'll fade into memory?

As I pack my hospital bag, I try to imagine what belongings might ease her misery. Will she be more comfortable in a sports or nursing bra? Will what's happening to her body make her overheat, or will she want sweats and fuzzy socks? Will she crave a robe or roomy pajamas?

What could I possibly tuck into my luggage to comfort this poor, traumatized person who has been battered and bruised, but must put her personal hurts aside and tend to someone brand new—this woman who is now a mother?

Letter to a Beautiful Stranger

Thirty-Five Weeks

To the woman in the Target checkout line who heard I was due next month and said, *"Wow, you look great,"*

God bless you and all of your descendants.

Sincerely,

Me

My Body Is a Big Fat Temple

Thirty-Seven Weeks

AT THIS POINT, I'M HELD TOGETHER BY CRUSTY GUM AND SHOESTRING.

Pain bayonets my back. My snoring sounds gas-powered (as I am). Constipation is so severe I occasionally check the toilet in the hopes that I gave birth. My crotch muscles are glaciers. Well, except for the leakage. Nobody speaks of all the leakage.

The degree of dizziness I experience is enough to cause windburn. Since I also happen to be starving, which makes sense since the baby is now growing half a pound a week, increasing his body mass like Christian Bale preparing to play Batman, I figure it might be low blood sugar and begin eating every two hours. For the first time in my life, I can argue that a brownie is for my health. I touch my belly like a mother goddess and murmur, "For the baby," with fudge lodged between my teeth.

The extra food doesn't appease the vertigo, so I call my doctor. I say, "The room literally spins for six or seven seconds at a time. I have to grab something to stay upright."

"I suggest you avoid places where passing out might be dangerous," she answers.

Doctors are so concerned with pregnant women falling, I'm surprised they haven't prescribed us training wheels, yet there's no attempt to pin down the source of my lightheadedness. Only in pregnancy, the grand mystery bag of ailments, where anything goes, do MDs hear such a range of conditions that they shrug at every infirmity, consider the preposterous normal, and don't bother searching for a cure.

They do want to see me a week later, however, when my underwear is saturated by what we assume to be amniotic fluid. If my water has broken, the baby could be exposed to infection. I rush to their office.

Don't worry. It's just pee.

• • • • •

According to my pregnancy app, my uterus has grown by 1,000 percent. I don't know why this is significant, but it feels worth mentioning.

• • • • •

We are out to dinner with some friends when all my muscles seize at once. My body is a broken-down jalopy. I pull off-road and ask Phil to roll me home.

• • • • •

I'm so fatigued, the workout video today isn't so much prenatal barre as prenatal lie on the rug and stare at the ceiling while everyone on-screen continues the routine. Yet, I'll soon perform the most physically demanding feat of my life, what I've been told is the caloric equivalent to running a marathon. I'm about as ready for it as Jim Gaffigan is to fight Ivan Drago.

My hands and wrists are stiff and swollen. Luckily, I removed my wedding rings so I didn't end up in the emergency room, weeping over two bands of gold sawed off my sausage link fingers. Despite ditching these marks of commitment, bachelors aren't tackling me on the street. Good thing, because my puffy ankles couldn't take the impact. Some women develop clown feet that never quite reduce. They have to invest in an entirely new pedi-wardrobe.

I've also acquired Popeye forearm, or what Phil affectionately calls Meat Paw. From the elbow down, I look like I could work at an Italian deli, crack open a Budweiser bottle without an opener, or shape horseshoes from raw iron. My prenatal masseuse actually asked if I was a welder.

Thanks to this inflammation, I can cross another condition off my pregnancy bingo card: carpal tunnel syndrome. Arm swelling squeezes the carpal tunnel and strangles the median nerve, a tangle of roots that runs from the neck through a wrist tunnel that really should come with hardier walls. Carpal tunnel syndrome is hereditary, as some people's tunnels are more accommodating than others. My mother had carpal tunnel syndrome in pregnancy and eventually required surgery. Apparently our line of carpal tunnels are skinny and get easily crowded, like the Lincoln Tunnel. Perhaps I should be grateful that there is *something* skinny about me, and that at least I'm not a passage-way from Manhattan to New Jersey.

The syndrome presents numbness in my middle finger, but rapidly progresses to tingling and aching in my entire right hand—which, by all appearances, could belong to Mike Tyson. Now my fingers are stiff and difficult to bend. I can't open a jar or hold a cup of coffee, so I lower my face and slurp it like soup.

As with most pregnancy ailments, there is no cure but delivery. I still have three weeks to go.

My body is a big fat temple, a holy place a squatter desecrated by making himself comfortable and practicing—by all accounts—his martial arts. Well, kid, consider this your eviction notice.

Letter to My Baby on a Day I'm Feeling Uniquely Meditative

Thirty-Nine Weeks

Dear Baby,

We're getting Penny used to your nursery. We bought a second dog bed and propped it in the corner so there's always a place for her. Sometimes we play audio of a baby crying and feed her a slow drip of kibble so she associates the bleats with something appetizing. I wish someone would do the same to me with chocolate chips.

We are communing in your room, Penny on her bed, your dad rocking on the chair with his laptop, and me lumbering around, taking stock of the changing table supplies. You're here too, of course, inside my beach ball belly, your foot or hand or elbow prodding my bladder. I can press my fingers just right and touch you.

You are a full-size human inside me: rolling around, crying, blinking against the light, listening for familiar sounds, flexing fingers and wriggling toes that I made. There are four hearts beating in this room I spent the last eight months assembling. We are breathing in and out, in and out.

The walls are cornflower and the furniture is gray. Three framed Harry Potter-themed prints hang above your crib. The mobile dangles four fuzzy objects over the place we will rest your head: a British-style bus, a taxicab, and two dogs. The clamp didn't fit over the rim so your dad secured it with nautical knots. You may not appreciate this yet, but that's classic your dad. Maybe, staring up at those ties, you'll grow to be a Gloucester fisherman. I hope, at the very least, your subconscious will absorb the essence of how your father cares for us in his signature way. Outside, snow pirouettes in slow motion. It's February in Massachusetts, and frigid. But it's cozy in here.

The crib is made with pinstripe sheets pulled taut. The dresser drawers are sorted by clothing size. There's a toy chest stamped with a blue-eared elephant and a laundry hamper embossed with a unicorn. There's a plastic garbage bag inside the diaper pail, poised for your deposits. A camera is hooked at the perfect angle and synched to view you at rest (or screaming wildly, as the case may be). A picture frame on the end table awaits your image. Board books line the shelves. Stuffed animals of all different genera—moose, frog, puppy, fox, and a couple of fantastic beasts—are scattered around the room, eyes beaded as a rapt audience. A cool mist humidifier is ready to be filled. We have diapers, wipes, and rash cream; sacks and swaddles; burp cloths, muslin washcloths, and receiving blankets; bottles, extra nipples, and pacifiers; spare sheets; a wrap and a carrier; a bouncer and a swing; hats, socks, and booties; a pack and play; and more onesies than you'll have time to wear before your limbs stretch out of them.

Everything is ready. We are here, and have all you'll need. We're just waiting for you, Baby. Just you.

Love,

Your Mama

PART V

Fourth Trimester

Labor Day

CONTRACTIONS BEGIN AT THREE IN THE MORNING AND ARRIVE AT IRREGULAR intervals—every eight, twelve, seven, fifteen minutes—like a train engineered by Salvador Dali, where clocks are hung out to dry. At first, the discomfort is a novelty, a challenge, and almost nostalgic, reminiscent of intense period cramps I haven't experienced in nearly a year. It's like being visited by an old friend. *Hey, girl!*

In the movies, labor is indisputable. Water breaks on a stalled subway train or deluges onto an irreplaceable rug at an antique store, or the contractions are tracked on a watch and grow closer together with increasing force. My experience is ambiguous. If you scatter-plot my contractions, they trend in the right direction, but there are frequent outliers. My doula suggests they might just be aches from the obstetrician going elbow deep into my vagina the previous day, twisting her hand around to break my cervical membrane, playing me like a puppet until I blurted out a safe word.

The contractions gradually deepen to feeling more like a boa constrictor squeezing my uterus, but they still don't converge into consistency. After a day without progress, I despair that this is false labor, another demeaning term. I have no idea if the cramps will continue like this for days or weeks, dissipate into nothing, or launch me into delivery. The uncertainty, and possible futility, is wearying. What if this day and half has been meaningless? What if this meaningless day and a half turns into three meaningless days, and *then* I go into labor, worn and dispirited?

102

I ball up on the couch and watch *Seinfeld*. Then, on the advice of my doula, I assume child's pose for thirty seconds and crawl around for five minutes. It feels ridiculous, but if it converts "false" labor into true labor so this isn't a waste of pain, I will howl at the moon. While George gets engaged, Kramer buys a hot tub, and Elaine is denied soup, I'm clambering around on all fours, as if searching for a contact. Phil comes home from work to find me weeping into the carpet. In solidarity, he lowers to the ground and crawls beside me.

After a total of thirty-six hours, contractions are five minutes apart (with outliers still), and they consume more of my attention, forcing me to clasp my temples or recede from conversation. The sensations hurt, but they don't double me over. I'm afraid if we go to the hospital, they'll take a piteous peek at my cervix and say, "Oh, honey. Did you think this was labor?"

Phil assures me, if they send us home, we'll just pick up Thai food and tell ourselves that's why we left the house in the first place. I go along with it, even though I have no appetite for pad see ew, which is saying something for a pregnant woman with two Nutri-Grain bars stuffed in every coat pocket. Especially since it's evening, and discomfort has precluded me from eating anything but a few scoops of yogurt and peanut butter.

My parents arrive to take care of Penny, and my dad snaps photos of me on my way out of the door, engorged as a tick and wincing. I hope he burns them or sells the images for use on an abstinence poster.

The previous May was apparently a spirited time in my town because the delivery ward is full. The hospital staff makes up a room in "the annex," which I imagine means rolling the mop bucket out of the janitor closet and wheeling in a hospital bed and fetal monitor. We wait on understuffed chairs and pray I won't be dismissed.

I gown, table, and let my knees drop in the manner that's become habitual. The doctor measures my cervix with what appears to be only her fingers and an OB-GYN Spidey-sense: 3.8 centimeters dilation. This is slightly disappointing since our doula suggested we delay hospital arrival until six centimeters, but it's enough that they keep me, which is enough for me. My body *was* gearing up for something these last days. This is labor.

Our nurse, a woman my age named Emily, says, "I'm on shift until seven a.m., so we've got plenty of time together. I want to meet this baby." Her lips open into a smile so wide it reveals the top of her gums. Brown hair is braided down one shoulder. I could imagine being friends with her, if she wasn't about to see me at my crankiest. I notice a nervous energy about her, a tremor below her open smile.

Thanks to Enza's lavender aromatherapy, we have the nicest-smelling closet in the hospital. She activates pressure points in my feet, calves, and thighs, using oils that stimulate dilation and relaxation. Her massages provide a pleasantness to focus on through the pain, since contractions are now every three minutes. She reminds me to slacken my shoulders, inhale into the contractions, and wash them away with a cleansing breath. She is a calming presence that sets an example for Phil. While Enza is stationed at my feet, he takes up residence at my head, stroking my hair, rubbing my neck, and admiring when the monitors reflect a contraction with an especially high peak. He carries a straw to my lips and whispers, "You're doing a good job. So good," with such sweetness and respect my eyes sting.

I take one bounce on a birth ball and decide, "Nope." I walk the halls, and when a contraction swells like an angry wave, I brace myself against the wall and Enza applies counterpressure to my hips. It takes us twenty minutes to reach the other end of the corridor. When we return to the room, she draws a warm bath and scatters battery-operated candles around the edges of the tub. I soak for as long as I can handle the increasing force of each contraction—about five minutes. It's beginning to feel like my uterus is being tied into nightmarish balloon animals until the rubber pops and the pain is released.

Our doula is not philosophically opposed to epidurals, but she does believe there are drawbacks: slowing labor; increasing the chance of a C-section; limiting mobility during labor, which compromises birthing positions; impeding the body's ability to push; and increasing recovery time postpartum. In her view, the ideal birth is epidural-free, but she supports the wishes of the mother. This mother wished for one all along, but hoped to hold off until at least five centimeters.

By the time I'm in the tub, I've been laboring in the hospital for five hours. If pain is a dial, the early contractions had been set at the lowest setting—period cramps, adorable in retrospect—but it's been cranked so that all my muscles clench and quiver for two minutes before they release, only to be strangled again in another two. I shiver to wonder how many notches of agony there are to go before the knob twists clean off.

I'm supposed to vocalize with deep grunts, but all I can muster is a pitiful whimper. "How far along do you think I am?" I want to be as dilated as this particular circle of hell. I want to have made it so I can quit.

Enza says, "I don't like to guess, but based on the strength of your contractions, I'd say seven or eight centimeters."

That's the cusp of transition labor, which is mythical in reputation. It's when wives say hateful things to their husbands. It's when it's almost too late to get an epidural at all. By her estimation, I am on the brink of feeling the ring of fire in all its natural glory.

"I'd like an epidural," I say.

"Even if you're almost there?" Enza asks. She hopes finding out that I'm close will motivate me to lower my head and sprint the last mile. It has the opposite effect. I worry I've waited too long.

"I want the epidural."

The anesthesiologist is called as pain rockets my blood pressure to 175 over 120. At the crest of every contraction, the baby's heart rate accelerates too. Enza and Nurse Emily shift me into different positions on the bed until they find one that satisfies the baby.

I thought hooking up the epidural would be an ordeal. In medical shows, it's a complicated and tenuous trick for new residents, and an uncomfortable one for patients. I scrawl away liability for possible paralysis before the doctor finishes his explanation. I'm boiling and can't see through the steam. I don't even register the needle piercing my spine.

My body quiets and the dread recedes. I've labored for five hours, plus the day and half before admission into the hospital. I've done good. I am in the clear. I won't feel the ring of fire. I relax.

The on-call midwife returns to check my progress. When I first arrived, she and the obstetrician introduced themselves. The OB inquired about my pain management preferences, and when I informed them I'd likely want an epidural, the midwife scowled and mouthed, "You won't need one." Now, as she assesses my anesthetized pelvis, I feel her judgment more than her finger. I anticipate hearing "seven or eight centimeters," as Enza had predicted.

"Four centimeters," she says.

In five turbulent hours, I dilated only a fraction of a centimeter, from 3.8 to 4. My mouth drops.

Epidurals often slow labor, especially when administered before five centimeters. I just increased my odds of needing a C-section, all because I couldn't handle the pain of early labor, never mind the active and transition stages.

I say, "I'm such a wimp."

Phil massages my shoulder. "Your contractions have been so powerful, there isn't even room for them on the monitor. The peaks fly off the charts. And they're coming one after the other. How could you *not* get an epidural?"

The doula agrees. The nurse agrees. The midwife digs her arm deeper into my canal, like she is reaching for keys she dropped between couch cushions. Warm water gushes down my legs.

• • • • •

Almost every appendage is hooked up to something. There is the epidural, the fetal monitor, the heart rate monitor, the blood pressure cuff, and the Foley catheter to drain urine. But the encumbrance of gadgets is a small price to pay to have Phil gaze over my head at the monitor and say, "This one is a doozy," and to luxuriate in the thrilling nothing.

Now that I'm not clenched with agony, my blood pressure lowers. I am feeling human again. We chat, of all things. Enza asks how Phil and I met, and then she tells us about meeting her husband. We joke. I eat cherry Jell-O and nap. Epidurals are witchcraft and I love them.

An hour later, Judgy McMidwife returns. Despite the reputation of the epidural, my labor has progressed. I am now six centimeters dilated. Whether it was breaking the water or being able to relax, we are finally cooking.

Two hours later, contractions murmur beneath the surface. I slurp orange juice and ask with the good humor of our mood, "Should I be feeling something? Because, it's weird, but I'm kind of feeling something."

Nurse Emily says, "As the baby lowers you'll start feeling pressure in your pelvis. There's nothing the epidural can do about that."

"That must be it," I say, and purse my lips to request another hit.

The pressure deepens over the next hour, to the point where Enza has to guide me through breathing exercises again.

"Are you sure I should be feeling this much pressure?" I ask.

"Is it in your pelvis or stomach?" the nurse asks.

It's hard to discern the difference between areas only inches apart. I say, "It's in the same place as before."

"I think it's just pressure," she says.

I consider that uncertainty I detected when I first met her, but suppress the distrust and click the epidural release button like it's a game show buzzer and I know the answer, but no one hears me.

• • • • •

The next phase of labor will be the barometer against which I compare all future pain. It feels as if I am being electrocuted every two minutes. I convulse. I puke up the blood of cherry Jell-O. I am tormented. The anguish is biblical: It's lepers who can't stand to be inside their own skin. It's the curse of Eve. It's back-arching pain, eyes-rolling pain. It's an exorcism. I turn to Phil and see his concern through the fractured glass of my vision.

Enza can't make demands of the medical staff herself so she types a message on her phone, telling me this isn't pressure. This is the full force of transition labor. I don't need a priest. I need the anesthesiologist.

Nurse Emily returns with the worst news of my life. The only anesthesiologist is in surgery; we have to wait another two hours.

I can't lie down. I can't sit up. I writhe. Every two minutes, when a contraction tightens, I despair, knowing it will crescendo into a vice grip, bulging my eyes and squeezing my soul from my body, before descending back into the new resting state of distress.

The fetal monitor strap shifts out of place mid-contraction and Nurse Emily leans over my belly to adjust it. I stare into the part of her hair while she fumbles. Something isn't working. Those nerves of hers surface; she tucks a loose strand behind her ear to get a clearer look. I try to give her time, I do, but all my cells are being wrung out, raked over coals, stretched and broken over a medieval torture wheel. Her touch is unbearable, and some part of me believes this pain is her fault. I push her hands away.

"I'm sorry. But we need to hear the baby," she whispers. I sympathize with the stress to fix this fast and get out of my way. Her fingers are working the monitor like a bomb disabler right out of bomb disabling school. I give her another ten seconds (or maybe half a second that feels like ten seconds) before I push her away again.

This pain is beyond the healing power of massage, pressure points, and scented oils. It's eating me alive. My body is a house on fire. The conflagration roars for one hundred and twenty seconds every two minutes for two hours before the anesthesiologist returns.

The last time the epidural man was in the room, I greeted him with a smile that contractions probably contorted into a glower, but it was, at least, an offering. Now I don't give a shit about courtesy. I don't even acknowledge him, but after taking his sweet time in surgery, he's lucky I don't reel back like a mythical sea serpent and chomp off his head.

Something had come disconnected; I wasn't receiving any of the patient-controlled epidural. The button I was pushing for relief may as well have been a retractable pen cap.

As he reruns the catheter, I am slumped and moaning, but conscious enough to hear Phil say, "Is that tube supposed to be squirting?"

I lift my heavy head. There is a leak in the new line and the anesthesia is spurting like a sprinkler.

"I've never seen that before. Must be a manufacturer defect. I'll just tape it up," the anesthesiologist says.

If I weren't on the edge of death, I would bring him to it.

The life being sucked from me as if by a Dementor is slowly restored by sweet numbing nourishment. My expanded lizard brain shrinks to make room for my human brain.

The midwife returns to check my progress. "Ten centimeters dilated. Ready to push?"

I'd made it all the way through the transition stage of labor without an epidural, but at least I wouldn't feel the pushing; I wouldn't know the ring of fire.

Phil assumes his place at my head. The nurse braces one leg and Enza braces the other. I surface from the swirling shadows left behind by the pain and ask Enza to remind me how this whole pushing thing works.

Every time a contraction rises, I am to lurch into a crunch, take a deep breath as if plunging underwater, hold it, and bear down into the pressure, pushing as if pooping for as long as that breath will allow, then take another breath and do it again and again inside the life of the contraction. (Of course women poop on the delivery table. They've been trying to do just that for three hours. Poop is the proof they've been doing it right.) After the contraction passes, I should relax for two minutes until the next one. Rinse and repeat for three hours, fueled only by a cup of yogurt and spoonful of peanut butter. If only I hadn't puked up that Jell-O.

I am freshly numbed, and have only a vague sense of contractions. "This is one, right?" The nurse looks to the monitor and nods. I heave up.

"Push like you're pooping. Push like you're pooping. Lower, harder. Give it all you've got, Mama," Enza cheerleads, my leg looped around her shoulder like a limb sash.

The midwife pokes around my canal and glares up my vagina as I grunt and squeeze. After a contraction, she drops her hand. "The epidural is too fresh. She can't feel her muscles. She's going to wear herself out with no result. We better let her labor down and try again in an hour."

I withstood the transition period all to be anaesthetized when I finally need to be in touch with my body. I received the second epidural at the worst possible time. What will happen if I still can't feel in an hour? How long will they let the baby hang out at the crest of the birth canal? After all that labor, will they have to do a C-section?

These concerns are nothing, though, compared to my gratitude for no longer being in pain.

"I guess I shouldn't have gotten that second epidural," I say, good-naturedly.

"You were so exhausted, you might not have been able to push anyway," the nurse says. "Besides, you're still having contractions even if you can't feel them. While you rest, your body will drop the baby into position."

I close my eyes and sleep for forty-five minutes. When I wake, we try again.

• • • • •

Three hours of pushing every two minutes comes out to approximately ninety minutes of crunching abdominals that have been hibernating for forty weeks, ninety minutes of holding breath, ninety minutes of flexing biceps into modified pull-ups, ninety minutes of force. I burst blood vessels in my face, probably my vagina too. It drains every ounce of everything I'm made of. I want to surrender, but there is no surrendering. This baby is coming out.

The head is butting my pelvic bone, but there isn't proof of progress, despite hours of work. I'm grunting and sweating and going redfaced as I strain. I can't fathom women who accidentally give birth. Nothing I've ever done has required so much active effort. If I can't navigate the baby over the bone, I might require forceps, a vacuum, or surgery. The clock is ticking, but its face is blank.

Enza reports that a tendril of the baby's hair emerged from the canal. I beg her to rip him out like a weed.

In the offbeat of contractions, Phil sticks a straw of ginger ale between my lips to provide energy and promises I'm doing a good job, though it's hard to believe. Whoever came up with the phrase "making headway" was not describing a crowning baby.

Enza reminds me to direct my power into my bottom rather than wasting precious energy clenching my face and shoulders. Nurse Emily flags particularly effective pushes and douses my labia and perineum with oil to minimize tearing, which I appreciate even in my disorientation. When I am too weary to lift my head into the crunch, she attaches a birthing bar to the bed.

It's the three of them lifting my legs and spirit for three hours. The judgy midwife pops in but leaves quickly. She doesn't even notify us when her shift ends and she goes home for the night. Nurse Emily is the only medical professional during the majority of the fifteen-hour process. Between contractions, she and Enza twirl the hair poking out my vagina, as if to offer Rowen encouragement too. His face is smashed up against a flesh wall, which can't be pleasant, but it won't be long now.

When I finally crest the head over my pelvic bone, Nurse Emily directs me to stop pushing until she retrieves a doctor or midwife. I cradle the great bulge inside my birth canal like a human sausage casing and wait.

Seven medical professionals file in and gather in front of the parted curtains of my legs to view the stage of my vagina. Modesty is irrelevant. Pooping in front of an audience is the least of my concerns. The star of the show is ready for his opening number.

The new midwife, who sees my labia before my face, introduces herself, but I don't give a damn who she is. I wouldn't care if the mayor walked in. Hell, I wouldn't care if *John* Mayer walked in. This is close to being over. That's what I care about.

When the midwife tells me to, I push like my uterus needs to move a tractor-trailer uphill.

People say pushing with an epidural isn't painful, it's only pressure. Tell that to the witch who was pressed to death. Pressure hurts, but there is so much hurt behind me, and I can see the end now.

If my math is right, freeing the head required around 135 sustained pushes. After two strong shoves, the rest of the baby's body dumps out of me in a deluge of skin and bone that cracks me open. I bellow like a mighty bull, or so I think. Later Phil will tell me I was silent. Maybe I only bellowed in my mind, or maybe Phil retreated into his own soundless universe as the woman he loves was torn in half and didn't hear her primal life-ending-and-beginning howl.

"Look up, Mama," says Nurse Emily, who stayed an hour past the end of her shift. Nurses ferry you through the most epic day of your life, and then you never see them again.

She carries our baby, a wailing purple blob with a goopy mat of dark hair, up from between my legs and places him on my chest. A glob of my blood beads across the bridge of his nose. He is still warm and moist from my insides, and he lays heavy on my naked chest.

"Oh my God. Oh my God," I repeat.

My hands grasp his rubbery shoulders. Someone drapes a striped hospital blanket and the baby's whimpering subsides.

This is the moment mothers describe their love as instant; they meet their child for the first time but recognize that they knew him all along. I crave that recognition as the badge of my effort, the emotional electrolytes that will replenish me after so much bleakness and exertion. I receive its absence like a missed step. Though this discon-nection is a small plunge, in its place, there is something else—an appreciation.

I don't know who this little person on my torso is, but we've both been through the ringer. He's only seconds old and has already experi-enced the most trying day of my life. We are fellow soldiers stumbling home. Or perhaps he's lifting a mirror up to my odyssey. Instead of seeing my son in his swollen face, I find a reflection.

· · · · ·

Mine was a typical delivery. It was of average length, I didn't hemor-rhage, the baby's heart never stopped, he wasn't in a breech position, I didn't require emergency surgery, they didn't have to vacuum the baby out or extract him with forceps, like tossing a stubborn salad. This was the run-of-the-mill finish, the bloody in-the-trenches, fifteen-hour-long trial women confront and don't publicize afterward, because it's too ter-rible to remember, because our stories aren't received with the awe and sympathy they deserve, or because nobody wants to hear it. Labor is an unhonored ordeal, even by other women—maybe especially by other women. My own mom rolled her eyes when another woman described her birth as traumatic. "She thinks hers was worse than the rest of ours?" (To be fair, my mother is a relentless one-upper. If you had a sore throat, she had strep. If you hit some traffic, she was at a standstill. Her tombstone will read, "You think that's bad? I'm dead.")

Just because childbirth is a universal and necessary horror doesn't mean it should go unsung. Mothers propagate our civilization with their sweat, blood, and tears.

And what of the partners in the room, bystanders to the torment, fearing what might happen to their families, trapped by helplessness? These experiences, too, aren't often discussed.

There will be much to come for my family—a placenta to deliver, a second-degree tear to stitch that will take three months and an in-patient cauterization to heal, a cord for Phil to cut, blood and fluids to pump out of my uterus by stomach CPR, fainting in the shower, icing my genitals, the miracle of the first bowel movement, hemorrhoids, weeks of bright red toilet water, lightheadedness and nausea, soreness, peri bottles and witch hazel wipes, and, oh yeah, a baby to raise—but for now, this small stranger and I already have one thing in common: we are so relieved to be delivered.

"Hi, Rowen," I say.

After all our deliberation to select a name with just the right measure of meaning and individuality, the woman in the next delivery room chooses the same damn one.

A Rant about the Husband's Stitch Which I Didn't Get, But Many Women Do

MOM IS WEARIED, COATED IN BLOOD, SWEAT, FECAL MATTER, AND AMNIOTIC fluid. Her newborn lies on her chest. She's just birthed a baby, and may birth another someday, but in between, she will have to please a man. She's a new mother, but still a wife. It's important to remember both of these roles.

The husband's stitch is the extra suture sometimes used to close a vaginal tear and narrow the opening. It is not a medical procedure. It is not provided with consent. The bonus loop is a wink at Dad, performed behind the curtain of Mom's delirium.

The extra stitch can make it painful for the patient to sit and walk. Sex can be excruciating for months and years to come. But that concern is secondary to the benefit enjoyed by the man. (Put aside, for a moment, that sex is best when it's best for both. It should also be acknowledged there isn't proof the husband's stitch benefits anybody. Perceived tightness comes from the tone of vaginal walls, not from the site of entry. Therefore, the husband's stitch is without any structural integrity.)

There aren't studies to track the prevalence of the husband's stitch in this country. It can't be numbered because it isn't recorded in files, as in: *Second-degree tear of the perineum requiring seven stitches and a husband's stitch*. The evidence is anecdotal.

We can shrug and call the husband's stitch a myth, a fable, a falsehood. We can say that women are mistaken who remember a doctor's wry remark or who live with hurt or who have different obstetricians unofficially confirm what was done. We can reassure ourselves that these mothers aren't wrong on purpose, poor things. They simply misunderstand the situation. They are in pain, but just suffering normal postpartum discomfort. Nothing out of the ordinary.

To say this would be easy, because it's easier to doubt women than to do almost anything else. And if we loosed this one brick, we'd have to disassemble the entire wall, and would find misogyny is insidious. It's mixed in the clay.

Feeding Frenzy

"BREASTFEEDING IS THE MOST NATURAL THING IN THE WORLD," WE SAY, BUT recoil when a woman lifts her shirt in public. "So much more convenient than formula," we say, while a mother holes up in her office bathroom as if snorting coke, balancing on a toilet with her pump battery on the paper dispenser. "So much better for the baby," we say, as the starving newborn who can't latch wails so furiously his parched tongue quivers.

Humans should have gone extinct by now. That's how hard breastfeeding is.

An hour after I deliver Rowen, when we are still on the bed soiled by blood, vomit, amniotic fluid, and, let's face it, feces, a nurse I don't recognize, part of the medical team that arrived while the baby was lodged in my birth canal and I was one layer short of being stuffed like a turducken, asks if I want to breastfeed. I've read how critical this moment is for bonding, and since I've dreaded being a defunct mother, incapable of proper attachment, I nod, thinking we both can use the hormone release. She paws my right boob like a hoagie whose fillings are falling out and stuffs it into Rowen's mouth. He sucks a few times and then unlatches. I will struggle to emulate that wild success for months.

Phil and I attempt to get Rowen breastfeeding in the hospital. With one flat nipple and one slightly inverted (Phil calls the trickier breast Old Lefty), there isn't anything concrete for Rowen to grab onto. It's like rock climbing without footholds. We toss the poor guy against the smooth mound and wonder why he keeps sliding to the floor. Well, he doesn't slide to the floor. He screams. And I continue

117

to mash my breast against his contorted face, hoping his squawking mouth will magically soften around my lame nipple and begin to drink. After copious frustration and tears all around, we forfeit and press that trusty nurse call button, saying pitifully into the microphone, "We can't feed him again." While there, the nurse conducts her magician's tablecloth trick to change my bedsheets so I don't wallow in my own blood and fluids.

Once, Rowen pulls away with a red drop on his lip. Only then do I realize my nipples cracked. I had no idea. Detecting one cut on my post-birth disaster zone is like noticing a single bullet on a battlefield.

Yet Meghan Markle, the Duchess of Sussex, stepped into the hallway of Windsor Castle two days postpartum in heels, wearing a *white* trench dress. There isn't a diaper palatial enough to give me confidence to walk in white. Two days postpartum, I'm either on the toilet or splayed on the bed, naked but for mesh underwear and the eagle wingspan of a maternity pad. Rowen and I wear mommy-and-me coordinated outfits, only he's wrapped in a blanket while I greet the cleaning lady who empties the garbage like Rose beckoning Jack. *Draw me like one of your French girls. Also, can we have more tissues?* I can't remember what it's like to wear a shirt, or that it isn't normal for people you just met to shake your boob rather than your hand.

Nurses and lactation consultants visit on every shift, each with her own breastfeeding method. The cross-body hold. The football hold. Tuck a rolled towel underneath your breast so it doesn't weigh so heavily on his chin. Hand express a bead of colostrum to get him interested. Aim the nipple to the roof of his mouth. Hold him tight behind the shoulder blades. Brace the back of his head. Press the top of your breast to make space for his nose. Be skin to skin. Massage him while you breastfeed. And massage the bottom, crest, and side of your breast—from the top down. No, up and inward.

The endeavor requires six hands, the most important stemming from scrubs. How am I to keep this kid alive without experts? Or, God forbid, by myself, when Phil goes back to work in a week?

It doesn't help that we're trying to learn this new skill when we haven't slept, I'm physically shattered, and my pelvis went eight rounds with a welterweight champ, but I barely manage to keep Rowen alive at the hospital. He loses twelve ounces. If he loses one more, we won't be able to take him home. I half wish for this, because I don't feel physically capable of even caring for myself—my head is a drum pounded by the mallet of a migraine, I'm woozy, feeble, disoriented, and my vaginal canal feels churned by an immersion blender. I don't trust my body to provide for a baby. Neither does the lactation consultant who meets us at discharge and equips me with enough accessories to build a bionic boob.

I am a breathing bruise and still can't walk without fainting, so they discharge me in a wheelchair, which makes me think, *You know I can't walk, and you know I can't feed this child, and you are pushing us to the door? Do the right thing, man! Let us live here!*

Most women don't produce milk for three days, which seems like an evolutionary disadvantage, but I'm barely producing colostrum, certainly not enough to support my nearly nine-pound turkey, who is becoming a heartbreakingly smaller bird by the day.

The feeding system provided by the lactation consultant works like this: a nipple shield—a silicone breast cap with an envious bulge—is stretched over my flat canvas to draw my nipple into the protruding cavity. Then we hope to rouse my desert aridness into a milky ecosystem via the SNS, or supplemental nursing system, which includes a syringe, feeding tube, and formula—enough ingredients to allow even Phil to breastfeed. We simply run the feeding tube through the top of the nipple shield, fill the syringe with formula, latch the baby onto the nipple shield, and dispense the formula through the tube at precisely the right rate so the baby keeps pace without getting frustrated.

See, what could be more natural than breastfeeding?

The idea behind the SNS is twofold. One, feed the baby. Two, stimulate my nipples through his sucking so they'll probably-maybe-hopefully begin to manufacture milk themselves.

It's a lovely theory but, in practice, the feeding tube interrupts the suction of the nipple shield, causing it to drop at the slightest upset and spew formula all over us and our bedsheets. Second, although the feeding line indeed pumps nutrients into our baby's mouth, it also pumps him full of air pockets, which produces enough gas in his little body to send him to the moon. He farts louder than Peter Griffin. Lastly, it just isn't sustainable. It's at least a two-person job. Phil and I both have to retreat every two hours—about ten times a day—to hook my breasts to this pseudo IV. Phil is going back to work in a few days, and I can't do this alone, so my milk production faces a deadline.

· · · · ·

My inadequate boobs are a topic of public conversation. Just as I'm collecting the dignity I scattered during labor and delivery, everyone is asking, "How's breastfeeding going? Has the milk come in yet? And what exactly is wrong with your nipples?" Even when dressed, I'm the only naked person in the room.

My mother, ever the sensitive passerby, takes one look at all my accessories and says, "How did we manage to feed our babies before all these contraptions were invented?"

I really don't know.

· · · · ·

Since it's hard to tell if any of my own harvest is making it into the nipple shield along with the formula, we monitor the development of my glands by also trying to pump or hand express. As any dairy farmer can attest, hand expressing requires technique. I'm not very detail-oriented or patient—I end up honking my boobs like a teenage boy, and when they don't transform into geysers, I decide my existence is futile. Phil, who teaches math to non-majors, knits, and feeds a sourdough culture on a daily basis, possesses the qualities I lack, so he, my husband, milks me.

"Is this weird?" he asks.

It has been a primal week. Hell, it has been a primal ten months. He was beside me as I puked, described diarrhea and constipation, grew hair in new places, shat myself, and leaked urine. He taped my belly and sprayed cooking oil on my wet, naked body when the adhesive blistered my skin. He timed my early contractions and encouraged me as I grunted through later ones. He soothed me and fed me sugary fluids for strength. He rubbed my shoulder as I barfed red liquid into a hospital bag. He watched an anesthesiologist administer two epidurals, pointing out when one was defective. He spotted the tendril of Rowen's hair poking through my vagina. He cut the umbilical cord. He examined the placenta. He changed Rowen's diapers when I was too depleted to move. He catered to me, swollen and aching. He was a rapt student while the nurses demonstrated swaddling and bathing, and while the lactation consultants manipulated my chest. Milking me feels about as ordinary as everything that preceded it.

The first pediatrician visit is two days after we leave the hospital. Through all the effort and aggravation of the SNS, Rowen gains back only one ounce.

"It's five days postpartum. If you don't get milk tomorrow, you aren't going to get it at all," the doctor says, with the gentleness of someone who treats children. "You've done all you can. Breast milk is better, but formula is pretty good too."

My commitment to breastfeeding was always flimsy, so I'm not anguished by its loss. What knocks me sideways is this: my inability to produce milk is physical proof that I'm not mother material. I may be nurturing this newborn, caring for him, rearing him, but not in the way only a mother can.

I worry that my body's shortfalls are a manifestation of emotional aridness. It's not that I begrudge Rowen; I'm devastatingly ambivalent. I feel as if someone handed me a baby, but not necessarily mine. I'm ready to care for him, but I don't feel a special, distinct connection. It more resembles early parenting reported by fathers. I lack the maternal bones. I'm just who I feared I'd become: a bad rat mom.

Phil and I continue the SNS overnight, finishing out three full days of feeding Rowen through four pieces of equipment, none of which is me.

I've given up on me.

• • • • •

The next morning, my milk crashes onto shore.

My doula, who has heralded the birth of hundreds of babies and the arrival of twice as many milky breasts, has never heard of such a late supply. I am a rarity. If we'd been in another century, in a time before formula and SNS, Rowen might have starved or been adopted by wolves.

After experiencing drought, I pump and hoard milk like a penny thrift who survived the Great Depression. The expensive electric name-brand pump draws on my nipples for thirty minutes without rendering a drip, but the twenty-dollar hand pump from a company called Haakaa, with a silicone grenade body and a trumpet head you squeeze and suction to your breast, yields at least two ounces from one boob while I nurse from the other. After each feeding, I measure and pour this liquid gold into storage bags, open the freezer to add it to my growing collection, and admire all my precious, precious treasure.

Once, when the pump loses suction and spills onto my comforter, I mourn openly. The brute who coined the phrase "It's no use crying over spilt milk" obviously never had to pump. Spilt milk is like spilt blood.

In his signature love language, Phil crafts me a rope harness with adjustable knots, and from then on I wear my Haakaa pump slung from my neck like a huntress with her powder horn.

Because I pump from one breast while I nurse from the other, I've tricked Old Lefty into thinking I'm feeding twins. Breastfeeding is a demand-supply enterprise. I begin to overproduce and wake in a tacky puddle, having soaked through overnight pads, a nursing bra, and pajamas. It's not practical to clean my bedding on a daily basis, so each night my sheet crackles beneath me. Breast milk pours down my stomach when I take off my bra. It drips onto the tile floor after a shower.

Each woman's nipple has fifteen to twenty openings. After days of a stalled engine, mine are now firing on all cylinders, and Rowen's tiny mouth has to tame this sprinkler head.

Nobody talks about how *loud* babies are at the boob. He gasps, huffs, and sloshes around my nipple. I half expect to look down and find him slurping a bowl of pho. Sometimes he goes quiet for a few breaths, relaxing, and the milk gets ahead of him. He throws his head back like a baby bird, but instead of worms, it's air he wants. Milk flows down his chin as he sputters and chokes. My overactive letdown is waterboarding him for information he is too little to have. After a few coughs, he blinks, stunned but otherwise all right, and returns to the nipple with a nose scrunch and headshake, his ferocity not at all diminished by what appeared to be a near-death experience. To keep him drinking in pace with the milk flow, I massage his shoulder like he's Rocky and I'm Mickey, saying, *You're getting creamed out there, Rock!*

Now that my breasts work as they were meant to (well, not quite; I still need the nipple prosthetic), people don't inquire sympathetically about the state of my boobs. Now they say, "Look at those chubby cheeks. Good job, Mama." The compliment is just as cringey as their concern was.

* * * * *

Breastfeeding is demanding and isolating. It's a mother's obligation, and since babies digest breast milk faster than formula, choosing breast-feeding makes the chore more frequent. I try to live life between feed-ings, but there just isn't time. For as long as I'm breastfeeding, which could be a year if I follow recommendations, I can't meet a friend for coffee, take a walk, have a beer—anything—without considering where I'll be and where Rowen will be when it's time for him to eat. I'm not a contortionist, so I can't manage the shirt lift, bra unclasp, nursing cover shimmy, nipple shield position, and baby latch in public. Therefore, my brain is constantly calculating milk math so I can get home in time. When they say a baby eats every two hours, that's timed from the *beginning* of the feeding. So if the baby nurses for an hour, you've got only sixty minutes before your boobs are back to bat. I'm the Cinderella of breasts. *If Rowen ate at eleven thirty then he'll need to eat at one thirty. It's twelve thirty now. That gives me a half hour to meet Amy for lunch and hurry back. Maybe if we get drive-thru my car won't turn into a pumpkin. . . .* Even if I pump in advance and provide someone a bottle with which to feed him, my breasts will still swell and need to be emptied.

This doesn't factor in cluster feeding, one of the many foibles you aren't warned about. Cluster feeding is when your baby wants to eat more frequently than normal. It might be every hour. Every half hour. You might be feeding continuously for four hours straight.

Rowen, for instance, is perpetually hungry from six to ten at night, and some mornings for the same hours. I Google it and read the blog of a lactation expert at a well-known national organization who claims this is normal behavior, particularly with breastfed babies. She says the recommended eight to twelve feedings (which, at thirty minutes each—best-case scenario—is six hours of feeding a day) is a minimum, not a maximum. When tracking how often she feeds her own baby, she once counted thirty-five times in a day. Thirty-five times isn't feeding your baby. That's wearing him as an accessory. I don't even like carrying a purse.

Despite getting milk, I don't feel like a more natural mother. My instinct drawer is empty except for some loose change and a detached button—wait, that's a spare nipple shield. I don't know what color the baby's poop should be. I don't know what his cries indicate. He doesn't settle in my arms. Pictures of us don't illustrate the primordial radiance associated with motherhood. I look like I've been sleeping and woke up holding an infant, having no idea how I got there. That's about how I feel.

I don't enjoy breastfeeding. Part of me wishes my breasts had stayed dry so opting out would be biologically decided for me. But the pressure to breastfeed is formidable. From the time I found out I was pregnant, a United Nations Summit of women, from my own relations to a random granny at a gas station, inquired about my intentions, or delivered leading-the-witness statements like, "You're going to breast-feed, right?"

There was the familiar singsong, "Breast is best." Or the slightly less irritating, "It really is better." Then there were softer encouragements: "Try it for at least six weeks," or "It gets so much easier after three months." But three months is a long time to do something hard when there is an alternative. Most people don't even diet for that long, let alone tolerate unproductive nipple chewing.

Research about breast milk is murky, observational, and often inconclusive thanks to confounding variables. Even studies in favor of breast milk indicate only minimal upsides, like two fewer diarrhea diapers a year (as reported by Emily Oster in *Cribsheet*), which certainly is not commensurate with the judgment flung at women if they don't continue a potentially difficult, burdensome, and lonely responsibility. Still, we turn our noses up at bottle-feeding mothers. (We'd also turn our noses up if they whipped out a boob, so maybe women just can't win.) We peg the powder mothers as uninformed, selfish, lazy, quitters. We lock formula behind glass at the grocery store like it's illicit, so they have to track down official personnel and muster up the courage to ask for the key.

• • • • •

There's a warm rope in my left breast. My chest has been engorged, leaky, achy, knotty, sore, cracked, bleeding, raw, and radiating for so long, I can't determine how abnormal this is. I press my fingertips into the end of the root and work my way forward along the braid. The pressure causes milk to spray from two nipple openings in a fine stream, like liquid spider's silk. I walk my fingers back and forth from the base to the crest—tapping, stroking, and kneading like a masseuse who specializes in boob, and wonder, briefly, if my divine masseuse does duct work, or if I should just call someone in HVAC—but the line appears connected to a bottomless keg; I can't drain it.

There are other ways I'd planned to spend my free time today, my precious free moments not spent breastfeeding, burping, changing, soothing, coaxing, and breastfeeding again. I might have cooked. I might have done laundry, or tried to take a nap. I might have finished up thank you notes for baby gifts, or—imagine—read a few pages from a non-parenting book. Now those fancies will be put on the back burner to address the machine of my body, and what may or may not be a clogged duct.

Online forums recommend soaking in a sitz bath, so I draw one and add to it the salt of a mother's tears, because now the obstruction has coagulated, or I've prodded my body too much. My breast is a hot spot.

We are due to meet friends at a brewery this evening, our first social outing with our baby, now five weeks old. I'm nervous but determined to prove we are who we were—we can live our lives!—so I give this bath all I have, soaking until an inch evaporates, refilling until our hot water heater spits fumes, and staying put until my fingertips shrivel into raisins.

I brace my body—my overworked, used-up, misshapen, hurting, healing body—on the edge of the tub. Water sloughs off me, and I am washed by a sudden awareness that I'm absolutely shuddering and so weak I can't hold myself up. I navigate my collapse over the porcelain onto the bathmat and whimper loud enough that I hope to be heard.

Phil collects me off the floor, wraps me in a towel, and shepherds me to bed, where he piles on every blanket in our closet. I'm a mound of quilts with a heartbeat, but I can't get warm. Phil takes my temperature—104—and feeds me Tylenol. I think, *Nobody is this sick without dying*. I try to contain my trembling. My teeth chatter.

It's likely this is mastitis, and since breastfeeding can loosen the block, Phil brings Rowen to me. It's excruciating to pull back the covers and expose my bare skin to the air. Phil wraps blankets around my shoulders while I position the nipple guard, but my fingers tremble it off course. I tolerate this polar plunge for as long as I can and then burrow back under my layered cave.

We cancel our plans for that night, but by then I don't care—I can't imagine leaving my bedroom, never mind going outside, drinking beer. Phil wonders if my brain is on fire, and debates bringing me to the hospital. We alternate pumping, breastfeeding, Tylenol dosing, temperature taking, and shivering before my fever breaks. When I step into the hall after being in bed for six hours, it is a tentative and shaky expedition, like when army heroes in movies step out of their bunker into the sunshine.

My fever persists at a low grade the next day, so I call my doctor and am prescribed dicloxacillin. The day after that, Rowen begins to scream.

Caring for a baby isn't easy, but Rowen's relaxed temperament has made it as easy as it can be. Now, though, he emits strangled cries of distress, like an invisible someone is pricking his delicate toes.

I call the pediatrician. The on-call nurse reminds me that babies are always changing, and he might just be entering a new phase of his personality. I want to say, "That's your diagnosis? He's becoming an asshole?" Instead, I mention the mastitis, and she snaps to attention. "But he's on probiotics?" she asks, rhetorically. Apparently my prescribed antibiotics could pass through the milk and mess with bacteria in the baby's gut, causing gastrointestinal distress. The OB hadn't mentioned it to me because, once out of the womb, babies aren't in their purview. It was my responsibility to check my medication with the pediatrician.

Stunned, I turn to the Internet and read the following on the National Center for Biotechnology Information website: "Limited information indicates that dicloxacillin levels in milk are low and are not expected to cause adverse effects in breastfed infants." That sounds dandy enough, except for the "limited information" part. The website goes on to say, "Occasionally disruption of the infant's gastrointestinal flora, resulting in diarrhea or thrush have been reported with penicillins, but these effects have not been adequately evaluated."

Um, here's a crazy idea—evaluate them. Adequately.

Probiotics balance Rowen's discomfort—hallelujah, he's not an asshole, at least not yet—and the residual aches and fatigue from my fever dissipate. There's no telling when and if milk will curdle into a clog again, or when Rowen's mouth will transfer an infection through my nipple and propel me into a feverish spin that takes a week to abate. I'm tempted to forego any future madness by throwing in the breastfeeding burp cloth, but the pressure to do right by my baby in the eyes of the world, and by my own standards, drives us back to my bed, our place, what I used to consider a dreamland for sleeping and sometimes sex that is now for feeding and sometimes sleep.

I keep at it—just for now, I tell myself. If I quit the task only I can perform, what I'm told is best for my son, what does that say about me? So I lean against a pillow and batter myself for not treasuring the preciousness of ethereal nesting, or marveling at my body's maternal demonstration. There are bouts of sleepy lusciousness, drops of honey I hold dear, but mostly I don't appreciate it. I don't, I don't, I don't. It's a lonely chore that spotlights where I should be natural but am actually hulking, bumbling. The whole thing is staged. Still, I keep at it. I carry Rowen into our milky harbor, where Phil and Penny float by but can never drop anchor, and I hope it evolves into kinship I'll grow to relish, or that I'm weaving a tapestry of nourishment I can look back on and admire, running my fingers over the strands that bound us.

• • • • •

Rowen's body is small, rosy, and curled like a kidney bean, wearing only a diaper, because anything more than that and the coziness conks him out after only a few swallows and I have to poke or tickle him awake to finish eating. When his mouth closes around the nipple shield, he grumbles and tosses his head side to side like an unruly mare, or like Penny enticing us to play with a stuffed toy, before quickly settling around the silicone, his furrowed brow melting as he sucks and swallows.

He experiences so many emotions through the course of one feeding, or at least that's what I perceive by his swinging expressions. There's the initial frustration before the milk lets down. After some delayed gratification, his eyebrows rise with each gulp, as if he thought the milk might be sour and is pleasantly surprised to find it sweet. Sometimes he liquefies into complete relaxation, and rests his cheek on his fist. When alert, he resembles a cartoon baby chimp from the nose up.

Through it all, we are stripped down, chests bare, skin to skin, heart to heart. I have nothing but myself. I am giving him all I have. He gulps it in big swallows, gazing up at me with those intense eyes and, in that moment, what little I have seems to be enough.

Baby Blues

WHEN WE PULL INTO OUR GARAGE, THE PUPA OF A BABY STRAPPED IN THE row behind us, I am washed by what feels like homesickness—but that can't be right, because after giving birth, our brand new family, all healthy, is returning from the hospital to our *house*.

It seems impossibly treacherous to carry the baby unprotected past rakes dangling from the wall, through the roaring furnace room, and up the stairs, so Phil lugs him in the upside-down helmet of his car seat, while I take account of all that is ours: there's the wooden wall art I bought in Brazil, there's the couch from Bob's whose springs snapped promptly after the delivery men left, there's the vase we found on our honeymoon, there's my dog, there are my parents. This is my house. My name is on the deed. I arranged the furniture, and it's just where I left it.

Everything is the same, yet painted with the unfamiliar, cast in a new light. I've stepped into a bizarro version of my life, especially that baby swing beside the bookcase, and the mew of the tiny creature in it who is apparently my son.

A stone plummets in my now empty middle, which is seemingly bottomless, because the stone isn't plunking against a soft riverbed, it's just sinking, sinking, sinking.

Phil clips a leash onto Penny's collar. She is thrilled to have us back, to be going on a walk, tail whacking the wall, but with each step they take toward the door, my air pipe constricts.

My husband feels like the only constant in my life. He can't leave me in this strange world. Only he knows what I've been through. Only he looks the same. I need him to stay by my side and to never leave me again. But what am I supposed to say? *Don't take the dog for a walk?* That's crazy. The door shuts behind them, and we are seared in half.

My parents—altered versions of them, now grandparents—scoop the baby from his seat and coo and marvel while I stand a couple feet back like an outsider. Though, isn't that baby mine? Where is my elation at having the baby out in the world, in front of our eyes?

I feel certain the only way to reconstruct any glimmer of happiness I used to feel, should be feeling, is if Phil, Penny, Rowen, and I move into our bedroom—better yet, our king bed—and never leave it and never let anyone else in, except maybe the hospital nurses, if they want to care for us as they so brilliantly did over the previous three days.

I can't reconcile my incongruence against my parents' delight, and can't expose that I'm feeling so lost when I should be feasting on this delicious infant, rejoicing in him, so I recede into my bedroom to prepare our future permanent residence, and cry as soundlessly as possible until Phil returns and finds me there.

"What's wrong?" he asks.

"You walked Penny," I say, as if that explains everything.

• • • • •

I am battered by squalls of despair throughout the first two weeks, occurring every couple of days, usually at night, lasting an hour or two. It feels like I'm dunked into a tank of grief. There is no escape hatch. All I can do is cry and hope I'll raise the water level enough to spill out over the top. I'll be managing fine enough, and then I'll feel myself descend, I'll sense the darkness closing in around the edges, and suddenly I'm grieving, grieving, grieving, and I don't know how to make myself better. These uncharacteristic bouts become so regular that Phil and I high-five if I go a night without tears, and then I secretly cry at how pitiful that is. When I surface, it's to a mood shades duller than happy.

I try to explain it all away—Phil is returning to work, I am tired,

I don't want to host—but the truth is, there is no explanation. I am just sad, and the irrationality scares me. It means I can feel anything anytime for no reason at all.

There is much to be happy about. I have a healthy newborn. Where I worried that Penny might show signs of aggression, especially since she isn't socialized to children, she licks his head like he is her pup. (Perhaps this is because my parents brought Rowen's delivery blanket home so Penny could sniff it, and placed it in his crib. Or perhaps, since my smell was all over it too, she'd assumed I'd died a bloody death, and was so relieved to see me again she didn't resent the loud shit-machine I brought with me.) Our family and friends send cards and gifts, call, text, and visit. My parents cook, clean, and help care for the baby. They snap photos of Rowen until their phones run out of memory. They analyze and appreciate him like two baby scholars. They loved him before he was born, and now here he is. A new child is a blessing, one so many other couples struggle to conceive. Sadness is not an appropriate emotion for a situation in which everything went right. I am not entitled to this feeling.

Yet, when I take a good look at our lives, Phil and I also resemble a family in crisis. There's spit-up-stained burp cloths draped over every chair, our bedroom smells of sour milk, half-drunk glasses of water are scattered like Easter eggs so that I can keep hydrated. Breastfeeding is a struggle that consumes most of my day. We hardly venture beyond the walls that enclose our chaos. There is a perpetual problem I have no idea how to solve, so we try everything: change, burp like this, rock like that, feed this way, feed that way, sing, pat, swaddle, wrap. We shower when we can. We eat when we can. We sleep when we can. But often I'm just staring at the clock, knowing he could cry at any moment, and my opportunity for rest is squandered by my own demands that I rest. This isn't the portrait of a young woman cradling her baby. This isn't pretty motherhood. It's wet and gritty and fierce. It's blood, milk, and tears. It's not knowing when darkness will yield to light. It's surviving.

My face, hands, and feet are still swollen from pregnancy. Now so is my vagina and perineum. My belly is a big, gushy, empty skin pocket, textured with so many squiggly stretch marks it looks like I've been lying on terry cloth. The once sharp stroke of the linea nigra that bisected my stomach from sternum to pelvis is now on such a soft setting, it points east until my amorphous cavern of a belly button and then quickly diverts west. Looking at my midsection in the mirror, I say, "My stomach is so gross." And Phil replies, "It's not *that* gross." So it is at least a little gross. My back hurts without the support of a core my fetus dropkicked, and my trapezius muscles are braided from craning my neck to ensure my breast isn't suffocating the baby. I haven't recognized the way my body looks or feels in a year, and I won't be able to reclaim it until another life no longer needs it to survive. I'm realizing that the phrase "getting your body back" doesn't mean restoring it to its pre-pregnancy shape, but having it be your own once again. I am still wearing mesh underwear and a diaper-size pad because I'm bleeding—a lot. All my clothes should be lined in that sacred mesh.

By the time my baby is only two days old, I've leaned on all the bad words flagged by good mothering professionals: epidural, pacifier, formula, and bottle. But I'm desperate. I'll do anything, because I don't know why Rowen is crying. Is he hungry? Gassy? Is there a hair tourniquet tied around his finger, toe, or penis? I reposition him and accidentally let his head flop a little.

He squawks in my arms and quiets in Phil's. It often feels like my baby doesn't like me, and certainly doesn't prefer me to anybody else, which doesn't seem fair, considering how much of myself I've given to him. His cells multiplied inside my womb. I felt his early movements long before anybody else. He slept with me. He absorbed my nourishment. I was the one to labor and deliver him. I should feel the most connected to him, and he to me. He should stir joy in his mother, yet every finger squeeze and head sniff that I anticipated to be a unique divine delight falls a little flat.

I don't leave the house. Home is where all his things are, and where no one can see that I don't yet know what I'm doing. I stay inside unless it's absolutely essential to do otherwise.

On one such unavoidable outing, driving home from the pharmacy, I pass through an intersection and will the car approaching from the left to stop, thinking, *I can't afford to die. Single parenthood would be too hard for Phil. Unless he marries quickly. Then it'd be fine, because his new wife will be just as good a mother as I am. It'd be all the same to Rowen. He won't miss me.*

It isn't a pretty thought, but it's not like I *want* to die, and I don't want to hurt Rowen either, so I assure myself this is just an unromantic (but accurate) view. It isn't postpartum depression.

• • • • •

Around the two-week mark, all four grandparents are in town to bask in the glow of Rowen. My parents visit in the morning and overlap with my in-laws midday, and then Phil's parents stay through dinner. They are all so eager to hold their grandson, I see Rowen only during the challenge of feedings before I pass him back off. I am a gallon of milk with arms and legs, and my spout doesn't even function properly.

When Rowen pushes himself off my breast that evening, I find an infant I don't recognize. His face is more oval than I remember. His eyes are wider and set farther apart. And since when does he have such a profound double chin? I am unsettled to find a strange baby at my breast, but we have company, so I cobble together my composure, thinking I'll just hold him for the remainder of the night so that I can relearn him, and memorize my boy.

I step out of the bedroom, and Phil's mother extends her arms. "May I?"

My in-laws are around for only two days. How can I say no? I hand Rowen to her, go directly back into my bedroom, and sob into a pillow.

Phil tiptoes in to say that dinner is ready. Given my mental state these last couple weeks, he isn't altogether surprised to find me shuddering in the fetal position. "Feeling sad?" has asks.

"Yeah," I say, without turning over.

"Want me to ask them to leave?"

I want Phil to carry Rowen in and place him in my arms. I want to see a baby I know. If not, I want to meet my son again. To learn him, and learn to love him.

"Just tell them I'm sleeping."

I know that baby on the other side of the door is mine. I held him while an umbilical cord connected him to the organ I created for his purpose. But when the cord was cut, the physical connection was broken, and a robust emotional one hasn't developed in its place, even two weeks later. I am fond of the baby. It is a defenseless thing I am responsible for and vow to protect, and I don't begrudge or fear that duty. I've been fulfilling that obligation for weeks: nursing, changing his diaper, cuddling him.

But I don't feel for him the way my parents seem to feel for him. They fight over who held him longest, spend hours gazing into his blinking face and laugh uproariously at any alteration in his expression. They burst with love, and their immediate attachment is a stark and shameful contrast to his mother's lukewarm sentiment. Why hasn't my love come as easily?

Since Rowen's birth, sadness has visited me as frequently as any well-wisher, but this time it brings shame and the dread that's been creeping on the edges of my mind since Rowen arrived: I don't think I love my baby in the way so many other parents do, when they gush, "We're so in love already." The love I'm feeling isn't unlike any other. It isn't immediate, unconditional, life-changing love. It isn't enough.

How can I love my baby when he doesn't even look familiar?

I cry for two hours straight. Then Phil and his parents exchange goodbyes and plans for the following day, and I meet Phil in the hall, my face red and puffy from so many tears. Rowen is balanced in the crook of his elbow, and he shifts the baby into my arms. I look down, praying to see an infant I can identify as my own, and choke in a gasping breath.

"I don't recognize him."

"What?"

I carry the baby to the bed where I've fed him eight times a day for ten days. If only we'd lived in this bed as I'd wanted, if only we never left and never put him in the arms of other people, maybe I'd know my son. Tears drip off my cheeks onto his striped onesie with the bulldog on the chest. I stroke his spiky hair and search his face.

"He doesn't look familiar to me."

"What do you mean? That's our Ro-Ro," Phil says, but there's a quiver in his voice.

"I couldn't pick our baby out of a lineup."

"Of course you could. You just haven't seen other babies lately. This one is distinct."

"It's like he's different from the last time I saw him, and now I don't know him anymore."

It's true that Rowen is growing fast and constantly changing. He's also so expressive, he looks like a different baby in various circumstances. He is one baby from my breastfeeding vantage point. He is another when he stretches in his sleep, elongating his neck and jutting out his chin like a chick. He is yet another when sleeping restfully, mature and a bit wearied. And still another when his eyes are open. They are dark, wise, and somber, drawing my attention like two black holes. Some expressions endear me to him. Some, like when he first wakes up and one eye squints like Quasimodo, make me wonder if he is even cute. (When I posed this to Phil, he answered, "Does it matter?") Sometimes he resembles a troll doll or Jon Lovitz. Sometimes, it's as if a persona drifts through him and pauses. Then it moves on, never to be seen again. I struggle to keep up, to know all of Rowen's many forms.

I should have learned him by now, but I haven't. I should have loved him by now, like other parents, like *our* parents, but I don't. Perhaps, as I delivered him, as my body broke in two, my brain also splintered.

"I don't know what's wrong with me," I say between gasps.

"You're just tired," Phil says. But moments later, as my cries soften and I rock Rowen, my husband pulls his laptop from the floor, glances to see if I will notice, and Googles, "Postpartum depression and mother doesn't recognize baby."

I don't mind; I hope he finds an answer.

While he scrolls and scans, I trace Rowen's hairline, bend down, and kiss his soft forehead. He smells like my baby. I close my eyes and inhale a full breath of him. Although my visual senses have failed me, there is sharpness in the olfactory. Earlier that week, I asked my dad to stop spraying his cologne because, after hours of him holding Rowen, Obsession for Men clung to Rowen's wild hair, overriding his more subtle infant smell. Losing that scent threw me off-balance. That smell was an anchor, and without it I drifted.

Phil reads symptoms of postpartum depression while I grasp Rowen's smell like a mooring. It grounds me. *You Are Here. This is your son. You are his mother.*

I relax into the milk and Cheerios essence of him, and other characteristics come into focus. He hiccups and I recognize that sound. He sighs his miniature wistful sigh. I know that sound too. I open my eyes, tentatively. He stretches his neck, scrunches his face, and resembles a hatchling in his nest, and I whisper, "I think I know that baby."

I set out to be a quick study, memorizing my son's features one by one; they are more consumable as standalones than a complete picture. There are his eyebrows, like fine sandy brushstrokes. His eyelashes, grouped in sparse collections. His eyes, like two oysters opening to navy pearls. His nose, flat at the bridge and propped up by two tiny donut nostrils. His lips, fuller on top with the bottom pulled in. His dainty point of a chin. From that moment on, each time I hold him, I recite his facial features like a mantra: eyebrows, eyes, nose, lips, chin. These landmarks root me in place while he shapes and reshapes into someone new.

My parents return the following morning. I need to speak this baffling, terrifying experience out loud in the hopes that I'll better understand it myself, so I admit how I hid from my in-laws, and how Rowen didn't look familiar to me. Tears spring back to my eyes, returning as if they had been waiting off-stage for their cue.

My mother comes forward to hug me. "I didn't have this as an Immordino," she says, referring to her maiden name. "We don't experience emotion."

My father, who is already cradling Rowen, presents him to me and says, "Look what you did. Look what you made." He pushes Rowen into my chest and reaches his own arm around me. "You hold your baby and I'll hold mine."

• • • • •

A postpartum pamphlet distributed at the hospital contains a two-sentence casual mention that 70 to 80 percent of women experience "the baby blues," defined as a fluctuating melancholy that peters out within fourteen days, possibly also involving mood swings, anxiety, fuzzy thinking, fatigue, irritability, and fear that you're not a good mother.

I'd heard of postpartum depression, but never the baby blues, not from friends or family, pregnancy books, or the doctors I saw every week leading up to delivery. For a condition a new mother will almost certainly experience, this oversight is disturbing.

As with most pregnancy-related issues, we don't know the cause, but it's likely the hormonal haywire of an abruptly non-pregnant body combined with milk production, the trauma of delivery, the stress of newborn care, and sleeplessness. When life undergoes an earthquake, there's bound to be aftershocks.

Sleep deprivation is particularly shattering for me. Before Rowen, I had a talent for securing ten hours of uninterrupted rest. Now that serving has been halved, sheared into fragments, and parsed. I dread bedtime. What used to be a peaceful drifting is now electric with anxiety. These aren't off-duty hours. Those don't exist. I'm at the ready, awaiting his cry, riled by the urgency to sleep while I can. For days, Rowen wakes every hour. For weeks, it's every couple hours. For months, it's multiple times a night. Between nursing, changing, and rocking, each bid takes an hour, and I spend another trying to forget the next call is around the bend. I don't know exactly how much sleep I piece together, but it isn't enough, despite beginning bedtime at seven o'clock. The dust of dreams undreamt clings to me. The expression "sleeping like a baby" should really be "sleeping like an adult without a baby."

Since we don't know the trigger of the baby blues, there's no cure, nothing women can do but soldier through it—the same sort of non-solution I'd grown sick of hearing while pregnant, and am discouraged to continue to hear postpartum—and pray it doesn't develop into a territory of concern, which is in itself imprecise to assess: When does a new mother's crying become excessive? How bonded is she supposed to feel with the baby? How happy should she be?

The line between normal and clinical is drawn arbitrarily, and not to do with the woman's mental health, but the baby's life. If a mother is weepy, we whisper, *Does she want to hurt the baby?* and if the answer is no, we exhale our relief and wave it away. *It's probably just the baby blues.* We feel comfortable allowing a woman to languish as long as, in her misery, she doesn't harm the child.

Throughout the first two weeks, I wonder if I'm experiencing good old-fashioned baby blues or the early stages of PPD. All I can do is wait to see how long it lasts. It does indeed endure past the mark, but milder, a spiked fever reducing to low grade, so it's hard to pin down the particular gray I'm stuck inside. Not wanting to make a big deal over my condition by making an early appointment, it's another month before I see my doctor.

Six weeks. That's how long the medical community lets a woman go without checking on her postpartum. The pediatrician examines my newborn three times before I meet my obstetrician. This, after the ordeal of delivery and complications of breastfeeding. This, after weekly appointments in the last months of my pregnancy. I couldn't shake medical attention when my womb was occupied, but as soon as I leave the hospital, I'm on my own for over a month. It begs the question: who exactly did they care about at those previous appointments if, post-delivery, I am cut loose?

Baby blues and postpartum depression aside, so much can go wrong in those first weeks. Over half of pregnancy-related deaths occur after delivery, even up to a year postpartum. Because of this, the American College of Obstetricians and Gynecologists advises that postpartum care should begin within the first three weeks and be an ongoing process.

First-time mothers outside the medical field, myself included, don't have any point of comparison, and would benefit from professional evaluation so as not to overlook atypical distress. A new mom could be bleeding profusely. She doesn't know if she's been pushing herself too hard, if she needs more rest, or if her discharge is normal. She doesn't know how much discomfort to expect, or if the aching is a sign of infection in her stitches. Or, if like what happened to my friend, she's allergic to her stitches. Or, if like what happens to me, the stitches dissolve before the wound heals. I assume the blood is from hemorrhoids and don't see a doctor for the prescribed six weeks, when they find an open wound and want to see me in five more, only to discover the wound *still* isn't healed and they cauterize it. My tear requires twelve weeks to close. I'm taken aback by the falsely advertised length of recovery, since everyone touts six weeks. The doctor says, "It's common to take much longer, but if we told you that, you'd never have children," and I promptly combust.

North of the war zone, women wrestle breastfeeding-related afflictions. Their nipples, used as utensils for the first time, are chapped, cracked, blistered, or writhing with a vasospasm. Their breasts could be engorged, the host to a yeast infection, or on the verge of mastitis.

There's also postpartum preeclampsia, deep vein thrombosis, hemorrhage, pulmonary embolism, heart disease, stroke, infection, sepsis, amniotic fluid embolism, incontinence, pelvic floor disfunction and hair loss.

Then there is the hormone imbalance below the surface. What can a mother do to combat the almost inevitable sadness, especially when exercising is limited because of her physical condition? When do those feelings cross into something that should be investigated and possibly treated? What is normal? Where is the support for new mothers?

Ten percent of the baby blues develop into postpartum depression. That isn't an insignificant number. Imagine how much suffering and shame could be nipped if depression was caught earlier than six weeks. All that time, women could have been enjoying their baby and flexing their new identity as mothers rather than hiding from family members in their bedrooms, staring into the face of their child as if they'd never met, wondering at what point their sanity fractured.

Postpartum depression is often depicted as a woman steering her car into a lake—a concrete and concretely threatening condition. But it's a spectrum, and there's an entire country of mothers who land closer to the baby blues, ambiguously despondent, set apart from their babies, scared, ashamed, and damp with tears. Their situations aren't widely discussed because they don't align with our perception of the hallowed mother, glowing with gratitude; because we worry they could discourage prospective mothers; and because their gloom is mundanely unpleasant—a bummer to hear about, without any of the compelling drama of a horror story. Or maybe we've just been convinced that the world doesn't care. The trials of new moms are icky, too irrelevant to public discourse—too female. We shouldn't surface such subjects with food present or, worse, men, who certainly have no appetite for it. So the stories of these women are kept behind glass, like store-bought formula; if we want to access them, we have to ask for the key. By not being forthcoming, we do harm to anybody window-shopping parenthood. Worse, we do harm to the world by telling less than half the story of motherhood

If we show women that we are hungry for their truth, that we want to listen, perhaps we can gather enough specifics that the topography of their suffering becomes clarified, and we can better discern when boundaries of normal yield to more troubling territory.

Most importantly, we the blue won't have to wander this terrain alone.

· · · · ·

Three weeks postpartum, my parents watch Rowen so Phil and I can take Penny for her first off-leash walk since the baby's debut. It is high tide in Beverly, so we go to the only beach that still has a stretch of exposed sand, which happens to be the same beach we visited eleven months earlier after the positive pregnancy test that would result in miscarriage.

New England beaches in March hold a certain bleak beauty. Wind cuts through fabric to chill skin. Crags beyond sandy inlets are snow-capped. The shore is unpopulated. In the summer, strolling the waterfront feels like vacation. But in the winter, you're alone with seagulls and shells that have been abandoned by sea life for other habitats. Braving the elements feels like an expedition, like you are uncovering an inhospitable frontier. Perhaps it is that spirit of exploration and isolation that kindles my courage.

"Is it okay that I love you more than I love Rowen?" I ask Phil. "He's my priority, but I don't think I love him yet, at least not above all else. Not above you."

The question rises off me like a noxious fume. As a mother, I wish my ambivalence wasn't so, and that Rowen had been immediately elevated in my heart. As a wife, I worry Phil has properly adjusted to parenthood, that my husband already loves Rowen more than me, and I'm suddenly the odd man out in our family.

I think of the night Rowen was born, after we'd been transferred to the maternity ward. I was resting (collapsed) on the hospital bed while Phil rocked Rowen by the window. Light strained through the edges of the blinds and burst around Phil's head. Rowen was wrapped into a baby burrito, and his new dad flattened his palm on his tiny chest and sang softly: "Some day, when I'm awfully low, when the world is cold, I will feel a glow just thinking of you and the way you look tonight." It's possible everything is clicking into place for Phil.

We amble on the beach while Phil considers my question and Penny bounds in the surf. Finally, he says, "You've only known Rowen for three weeks. We have a ten-year history. It actually sounds pretty natural."

"But other people say they fall in love with their kid immediately."

"That's what they *say*. Even if it's true, that's other people. You've never been much of a romantic." He whistles for Penny and feeds her a treat. She scarfs it down and scampers back to the water.

I think back to when we adopted Penny. Phil went gooey from the moment she licked his chin, but it took me months to form that connection. She was a floppy puppy I liked to play with, but she was also work I resented, and sleep I lost. She didn't feel like an integral part of our family until that moment when I discovered her distressed, tied up in her lead. Only then did something snap into place in my brain, and loving her became instinct rather than intention.

Phil continues, "If it makes you feel any better, I'm not overly connected yet. He's kind of boring. But our attachment will develop with rapport. Think of how much you've learned about Rowen in just three weeks, and how those small glimpses of his personality have made you more attached. It's only going to grow."

It's true. As the tide of my sadness recedes, Rowen and I are doing our own version of courting. I am getting to know him: When sleeping in my arms, he rests his cheek against his hand like a Gene Wilder meme. When energetic, he pinwheels his arms, just like he did in that first ultrasound. When he's drunk his fill, his body slackens into pudding. His eyes flutter closed when we're washing his hair under the faucet, like mine do at a salon sink. When he gets a pacifier, it bobs in his mouth and he clutches both fists at his heart. When he's pooping, he puckers his lips into a tiny Zoolander knot. His eyelids grow heavy when his Samsonesque hair is caressed. He is a trooper, usually only crying when hungry, cold, or especially gassy. He weathers even the most relentless case of hiccups and sits without complaint in a dirty diaper. It's as if he knows I need help and is doing his part to be easy.

If I'm going to live with myself, I have to accept that love is not simply going to arrive for me. And maybe that's no surprise. I've always lagged behind my peers. I didn't get my period until I was fifteen and I didn't start *The Office* until season six. The progression into mother-hood hasn't been easy or automatic either. Not the decision to have kids, pregnancy, labor, delivery, producing breast milk, feeding, or car-ing for a newborn, so why should this part be? And anyway, I'm not interested in easy or surface love. I want love that is gathered—sturdy, complex, and layered love that calcifies into something unconditional. I want the love of knowing someone. So I have to be patient. I have to give our relationship time to develop: slow, but made of solid stuff.

As I am getting to know Rowen, he is getting to know me. Scarier still, he is getting to know the entire bright-loud-hot-cold-crazy world he tunneled into. It's my job to show him that he can trust me, that I'll keep him safe, and to be his guide to all the wonders of this some-times scary but often hopeful place. I can do that.

As we arrive at the end of the beach, Phil adds, "Anyway, you do love Rowen. I see it. It's just not yet in the way you imagined."

I consider this point. Maybe I am doing just fine as a mother, and the only way I am falling short is of my own expectations.

⁕ ⁕ ⁕ ⁕ ⁕

After feeding Rowen in the still and shadows of two in the morning, we rock on the glider in his nursery. It's just him and me—we might be the only two people awake in the neighborhood—illuminated through the window by streetlights and a slice of a waning winter moon.

Rowen is fussing—he wriggles on my lap and his mouth stretches in pain. I coo my sympathy and rub his belly, the way I like my upset belly rubbed. He is the only person I'd coach through constipation.

As I soothe, his expression softens and his big eyes, whose dark irises have burned through cloud cover to reveal their dynamic blue granite below, fix on my face. Suddenly, he grips my fingers, one hand vising my thumb and the other my pinkie, and pulls my palm against his stomach, as if to emphasize that he wants me there with him, as uncertain as I've been. My face, worn and unsure, is reflected back to me in his pupils, and what I find there looks a lot like love.

Letter to My Future Self

Dear Future Me,

By now, your body has brainwashed you.

Pain memories are a biological imperative that is key to our survival. We remember what has harmed us so that we may avoid those things, thrive, and, ultimately, reproduce. A shutter button snaps in our brains to make permanent the fear of everything from a hot stove to braving a snowstorm without gloves. Everything but childbirth. A clear memory of labor and delivery would discourage women from propagating the species, so hormones are released to wipe the slate clean.

Future Alena, listen to me: During pregnancy you vomited, your muscles froze, and you grieved. During labor you clenched, you convulsed, and you grieved. Postpartum, you passed out, you leaked, and you grieved. It wasn't pretty. Don't do it again. Especially since, the next time through that ordeal, you'd have an existing child to think about.

Rowen will be staggering through his first drunk dinosaur stomp-walk when a well-intentioned birdbrain will ask, "So.... when does he get a brother or sister?" And who knows, by then—nine, eleven, thirteen months from now—you might be tempted. You might be missing the time before your kid could say no. You might feel pangs for baby yawns and thigh rolls. You might—heaven forbid—even be nostalgic for the intimacy of breastfeeding. You might be asking, "Was having a baby really that hard?"

Yes, yes it was.

You just don't remember because you've been hit with the hormone equivalent of the Men in Black *neuralyzer. Your brain has been shaken like an Etch A Sketch. Time has sanded agony's memory like tides erode a cliff's edge. It's no surprise that science still doesn't understand how, when, or why we undergo this convenient forgetting, but studies show we do—or at least 50 percent of us do.*

You might be persuaded to give procreation another go by women who glamorize the experience. They talk of the radiance of pregnancy, and how empowering it is to create human life. They liken pregnant women to holy Madonnas, except I don't remember reading a passage about the Blessed Mother shitting her pants. For you, pregnancy wasn't so much a celestial experience as it was a foray into the life of a long-distance trucker who ate bad roadside meat.

Labor and delivery wasn't any more deific. You weren't in awe of the process, as your mother-in-law attested to being. You didn't savor every sensation, like one of your natural-birth Facebook friends reported. The "sensations" were enough to make you want to detonate. Just explode, right there on the hospital bed, hopefully taking out the self-righteous midwife with your blast.

*So much suffering for a life in which you hunch over to collect milk as it drips off your nipples like Harry Potter phoenix tears. For saying sayonara to an uninterrupted night's sleep, maybe for years. For perpetually having a load of laundry to wash. For getting pissed, puked, and pooped on, all before noon. For sacrificing your body. For the bang-your-head-against-the-wall tedium of a baby's needs, because infant cuddles are sacred salves but, after a while, also kind of boring. For trying to understand someone who is irrational and random. (*What does it mean when his mouth takes that shape? What does it mean when he squawks in that pitch? *He's a baby. It means nothing.) For stuffing food in your mouth with one hand while the other peels back a diaper edge to see if that fart was wet. For crying, crying, crying (one for Baby, one for you, and one for when you're crying together).*

When you complained about women having to operate as normal in their last trimesters—commuting to work with back pain, sitting at a desk with back pain, smiling with back pain—your mother, sounding eerily like a 1950s adman, said, "Back in my day, you didn't work late into your pregnancy. This is what women get for having it all."

Well, "having it all" doesn't end with pregnancy. Post-delivery, you continue to have it all: Sexual desire and vaginal pain. Wishing your baby was a more restful sleeper and rushing to his crib when he finally quiets. Insomnia and dozing standing up. Loneliness and an aversion to socializing. Guilt and resentment. Peace and anxiety. Joy and sadness both.

I wince at the idea of having sex again, and not in the way of that classic sitcom joke in which wives are averse to having sex with their husbands. I like sex. But I'm literally frightened to put anything in the place a baby so recently burrowed out from. A doctor's recommendation for the first attempt was "Lubricate and inebriate," which sounds a lot like what Aunt Lydia might advise a handmaid.

This is what you want to do all over?

Women who recall the unpleasantness of childbirth promise the ends justify the means. If you are going to fall prey to one argument, it'll be this, because it at least acknowledges the truth that creation kind of sucks, and counters with your son, who would not be possible without such a trial.

Well, Future Alena, I don't know about the kid you have, but I'm with a five-week-old version who doesn't respond to my gestures of love. He might recognize my face and smell, but only as a food delivery system, the way you recognize a storefront as a pizzeria and are suddenly starving. Whenever I hold him, he roots and fusses, even if he just ate. We can't ever just hang out—nuzzling, cuddling, or simply being still together—like he does in other sets of arms. If he's with me, he wants to eat. He cares about my body and nothing else. It's the original form of female objectification. It's easy to feel used in this dynamic, especially when he's content elsewhere. I'm supposed to love this thing who can't see me past the tip of my nipple.

This morning, I just couldn't please Rowen. I stroked and rocked him. I swaddled and swayed. I shushed and cooed and whispered in his ear. He'd just eaten, so he couldn't be hungry, but I fed him anyway: right boob, Old Lefty, and then a bottle. He wailed through it all. Exasperated, and desperate for quiet, I passed him to Phil. He settled almost immediately, and I burst into tears.

"He's just a baby. He doesn't make sense," Phil said. "It isn't personal."

Yet nothing in my life had ever felt so personal.

Now Rowen is content, lolling in his bouncer, where he has been slumbering for two hours while I work, keeping me company, I guess you could say, his hands loosely circled around plastic rings on the seat strap between his legs.

That's actually pretty remarkable because he's sat in this seat every day for weeks and has never held the rings before. He didn't seem to know they existed. Maybe that's a sign that objects will soon begin to engage him. I wonder how I'll feel when he can interact with me, how our relationship will evolve when I'm not just a pair of breasts with arms and legs, but Mama, a person.

He's turned his head so that his chin rests on his shoulder. Each exhale is a gentle sigh. As I watch, his arms jerk in front of him, fingers splayed, like a baby Frankenstein's monster, and then they relax and float back to his stomach. This is the Moro reflex, a healthy sign that his nervous system is developing. Still, it's a little pitiful knowing he's startled by the sense of falling out here in the vast world that is so different from the tight womb to which he was accustomed. His flinch is followed by a big sleepy stretch and adorable grunting. His eyelids part just enough to reveal two slits of deep blue, and there is a tug at one corner of his mouth. It's not quite a smile, but maybe soon it will be.

Rowen is beginning to resemble Phil around the nose and mouth. His eye color could always change, but right now his irises are rich and round sapphires, like his dad's, and I find myself gazing into them the way I used to admire Phil's back when we had time for such things. I always knew Rowen could end up looking like one or both of us (or neither), but I didn't fully comprehend what it would be like to watch the similarities emerge.

After Phil passed the baby back to me this morning, Rowen's howls started up again. I finally calmed him down by singing Fleetwood Mac's "Go Your Own Way." I didn't remember the verses so I sang the chorus forty times in a row until he fell asleep. This tells me he's like his dad in two ways. One, he's a fan of classic rock. And two, he's the kind of guy who won't complain about lunching on a PB&J every day for the rest of his life.

But remembering my floundering Stevie Nicks also reminds me that the baby does in fact respond to at least some my efforts—maybe not always, or when I think he should, but he isn't completely impenetrable. He knows I'm there with him. Yes, he associates me with meals, but is it all that surprising that he's made such an association, given the limited exposure of his lifetime? He'll make more connections every day, but for now, he forces me to be creative, to dig deep, to mix it up. He hears me when I sing. Every day contains countless failures, but also bursts of these small triumphs.

In the same way Rowen challenges my perception of this morning, he casts my pregnancy with a different sort of haze, because only in retrospect do I appreciate that he was there in the fog, sweet and curious, through every bout of nausea and every bodily ache.

Rowen might be the story that revises me, forcing me to reconsider all that's happened under the light of retrospect, and apply those revelations to everything that is to come, and if I've learned anything in my life as a writer, it's that each revision is an excavation, an evolution, an unfolding. It bolsters the heart. It expands and refines a living breathing thing so that what was once thought to have merit in its own right is cultivated into something more profoundly multidimensional. The process is as confounding as it is dazzling, a beautiful catastrophe, but when it's finished, you emerge improved. And that's what happens with a sentence, a narrative. Imagine the phenomenon with a walking, talking, dancing, rejoicing creation—a work of art.

Shit, you're going to do this again, aren't you?

Sincerely,

Past You

PART VI

The Rest of the First Year

(well, not so much rest)

Bodies in Motion

ROWEN IS TUCKED AGAINST ME, HIS PUDGY CHEEK ON MY SHOULDER, HIS breath warm and wet on my collarbone, smelling of milk, his feet up near my belly button. I stroke the wrinkle of fat at his wrist and the dimples of his knuckles. His skin is cream satin.

I bury a kiss in the thicket of his hair, which was the talk of the maternity ward, remarked upon by every nurse, pediatrician, lactation consultant, medical assistant, administrator, midwife, obstetrician, food service and housekeeping professional who entered our room. Although it has lightened, it began like an Elvis toupee. Despite its bronzing, it often appears darker after grandparents and other visitors run their fingers through it, caressing goose down over a velvet scalp. They can't help themselves; it is so incredibly delicate. Such softness is rare in this world, and fleeting. We are quickly hardened, weathered, made coarse and gray. We pet him and our oils sculpt his locks into pliant hedgehog quills. My older brother Greg, who fears that his own hair is thinning, says the sheer volume is a gift wasted on the young.

Many newborns lose their hair within the first six months, after a hormonal plunge—the same reason women grow luxurious manes during pregnancy only to tragically slough it in handfuls once the baby is expelled. What will happen if Rowen loses his most defining feature? What will people say when they see him, if they can't say, "I've never seen such a head of hair"?

So much about him is already changing: The cord that connected me to him was severed, and its stump shriveled, blackened, and fell off to reveal a fresh belly button. (The dead detritus repulsed my younger brother Ryan so deeply I nearly boxed and mailed it to him.) The foreskin of Rowen's penis was clipped to expose an angry red head whose temper has since cooled. The lump from where his crown confronted my cervix has flattened. His features have defined as the swelling of delivery reduced; he no longer sports a mole snout or chipmunk cheeks. He shed lanugo hairs on his ears and shoulders, but has retained a tuft on the small of his back to match his dad's.

He'll continue to mature, and then, though it's nearly impossible to fathom, when he's here long enough—God, let him be here long enough—he'll degrade. His bones will harden only to break. He'll grow tall only to hunch. He'll learn to run, and then he'll ultimately slow. Nuzzling him in bed, I feel like a sleepy Mufasa, without any of the bravado imbued by James Earl Jones. *You'll feel indestructible, and then you'll learn how vulnerable you really are. That's the circle of life, kid.* As soon as he left my body and entered the world, he became subject to the elements, the way we all are, the way I sure as heck have been.

Rowen wears only a diaper, but blankets and my own body warm him. My finger traces the crook of his elbow. Does he sense that my finger is rougher than his skin, dried from sun and wind exposure, toughened from shoveling snow, cooking, lifting weights, and typing millions of words? Does he want to recoil at my touch, or is the difference mysterious and intriguing? Does he associate this particular brand of callous with his mother?

Maybe one day my body, no matter its condition, will impress him, since its most recent disrepairs are a result of growing him from scratch. Without having to think about it, I formed his fingernails, earlobes, and kidneys. I wired a nervous system when I can't even puzzle out our Internet router. I assembled body parts I don't have myself. My body's ability was nothing short of miraculous, but it wasn't a free service.

I now appreciate why Catholics make such a big deal over the Holy Mother. Sure, God sent His son to earth. That was an act of love. My parents had a hard enough time when Ryan went across the country for college. But Mary did the truly hard bit: unwed and swelling by the day, carting her tremendous belly across the desert by donkey, probably barfing into the sand and definitely spewing fluids into the grungy stable hay without painkillers more sophisticated than a horseshoe to bite on so as not to disturb the snooty guests at the sold-out inn. God bless her.

My body will never be the same as it was before. The act of creation transforms the creator. Stretch marks will remain like a forest of tree branches across my midsection. Scars from the kinesiology tape will fade but never disappear. Looseness around my belly button may shrink, but my tummy will forever feel empty after knowing full. My breasts will always hang longer and lower after months of acting as lunch bags. My pelvis will remember what it was to open to ten centimeters, to push out a body that was small, but not small enough to ever forget.

I'll never be a person who hasn't carried a baby to term, who didn't labor actively for fifteen hours and push for three. How could I expect to be the same person I was prior to such an event? When I looked in the mirror before pregnancy, I didn't expect to see a younger version of myself. Over the years, my jaw jowled, lines etched across my forehead, my middle softened, and my thighs dimpled. I have accepted those physical adjustments, and I'll accept these new ones too. Pregnancy was a sharp veer onto a one-way road with a higher speed limit.

This is who I am now—worn, wizened, and a little saggy. I'm on the downward trajectory, losing the very vitality Rowen's unscathed form is only just approaching. But I am not alone. The cost of living is high, there aren't any discounts, and we are billed too soon. This is a universal truth.

My Father

Before I was born, my father played street hockey in Forest Park in Queens, New York, and then he and his friends drove the Long Island

Expressway in the pitch of midnight to an ice rink. There he worked his arms at his sides and raced toward the puck, the chill and his exertion rosing youthful cheeks. He didn't care that there was a long drive home or that he had to be up for work in several hours. There was only that moment, all neurons firing, young and completely alive.

When we were kids, he wore muscle shirts and spandex leggings while he sold computer equipment remotely, intermittently descending into the basement to lift weights or work out on his motorless NordicTrack ski machine from the 1980s, with arm pulls and leather foot straps. Some dads fished. Some read. Mine flexed and called his biceps "the Pythons."

Rheumatoid and osteoarthritis sprouted when he was fifty years old. No matter how he yanked and sprayed, the weeds grew faster and stronger: Twenty-five surgeries, many that failed or worsened his conditions. Hospitalizations. Appointments with doctors of every specialty. The Mayo Clinic. Drug trials. All the medications. Yoga. Acupuncture. CBD oil. Soaks. Diets. Rest. Exercise. Stretching. Fasting. Praying, praying, praying.

Who we are is so dependent on how we feel. When I was pregnant, nauseated and then in pain, I was still myself—I wrote stories, watched sitcoms, lived for soft serve—but it changed me too. My humor became more pointed. I read books I wouldn't have before. I cared about new issues. I was treated differently based on my appearance, afforded some courtesies, asked particular questions. But I also missed out on certain conversations in favor of maternal ones, or was left out of plans. Pregnancy made me both more approachable and more isolated. In those ways, I was, as several people described, "all belly."

There were moments when my body didn't seem like my own, when I felt disconnected from the strange and constricting vessel carrying around my true self. At least pregnancy is temporary. Mostly, anyway. It's a complete body renovation, but then you're somewhat restored, save for a few modifications. Aging is permanent, so we mourn what we once knew, and what can never be again.

Tucked into the mirror of my father's dresser is a photo of his younger self wearing a hockey jersey. I imagine he gazes at that image when pain awakens him at night, remembering how it felt to be twenty and spirited, when his mustache was thin and the bangs of his 1970s hairstyle fell into his eyes, when he lived to roll and glide until his breath quickened and he felt his young heart beating in his chest. When his only limits were boundary lines.

My Older Brother

Greg has practiced capoeira, a Brazilian martial art that disguises self-defense as dance and acrobatics, for twenty years. His body is an expression of a different culture, and a nonverbal way of communicating with another person.

In capoeira, the point is not to strike, but to have a conversation made of attacks and dodges. Bodies fully engage in the present, responding to one another, rising and falling like interactive waves. The goal is to make yourself fluid, to flow through the collaboration seamlessly. If your partner stutters, you are meant to control your force, halt the flow, bite your tongue.

Kicks are circular or direct, toes pointed or flexed, each spoken with different intonation. Hand strikes are rare, but when uttered, they mean something. There is ground movement, balancing on wrists, elbows, and heels. Because sometimes people shout, there are also showier exclamations. Takedowns and flashy acrobatics make passersby eavesdrop. But so does speed.

How did my parents watch a stranger's heel whiz by their son's nose, touch the ground, and flash back to his precious cheekbone, or as their baby's own two feet sent him airborne? There are enough dangers in this vast unknowable world before our children invite strangers to almost hurt them.

This, I imagine, is how a heart is altered, tenderized, by parenthood. It's pushed to the edge of a precipice, forever on bated breath.

How does one survive it? I pull Rowen close and whisper, "No martial arts. Only chess. Acrobatics of the mind."

A year before Rowen was born, while performing capoeira in front of an audience, Greg did a routine backflip. It might have been his three hundredth, his thousandth, but this time, when he landed, his Achilles tendon snapped.

A doctor in the crowd helped him offstage. "Achilles tendon ruptures are serious," the doctor said. "You'll never be the same."

Greg wasn't ready to be changed. Over the next few days, he searched for surgeons who catered to athletes, who could make him the same again.

I drove him to the consultation an hour away. We listened as the orthopedist described the procedure and the intensive recovery: begin bearing weight six weeks out of surgery, return to activity after six months, hope for full recovery by a year.

Six months without capoeira. It was like telling him he couldn't speak for that long.

Greg's neck reddened, his veins were ropy. He coughed to steady his voice. "But the gymnastics. I might be able to do them again one day?"

The doctor nodded. "It's possible."

He waded through immobility and learned to walk again. Now he eases through milder acrobatic moves, but hasn't endeavored the full impact of a flip, remembering the way his body snapped doing what it had done so many times before.

My Dog

When Penny runs, it is with abandon. Across beaches, fields, and woods, her hind legs thrust backward and her front paws reach. Her muscles undulate beneath glossy fur. Long ears and a taffy tongue bounce as her feet dig and launch her back into flight. She looks at us with a grinning muzzle that says, *Friends! I'm running!*

At a local canal, we walk the embankment one mile down and one mile back while she takes the route by water, occasionally turning to confirm she is keeping pace. There are at least ten other dogs off-leash. Maybe half wet their paws. Maybe half of those fully immerse to retrieve a ball. She is the only canine paddling for pleasure. Onlookers comment, "She sure likes to swim," or "That's quite the Michael Phelps you got there." And we smile and nod like proud parents who don't want to boast, but what we're thinking is, *She's our phenomenon.*

We first noticed a swagger when she was a year old, after she'd been tackled in conservation land by an exuberant hulk of a dog, too eager for play. In the midst of their somersault, she yelped.

We rested her. We brought her to the vet, who assured us it would heal on its own. We walked her with a chest harness. We administered glucosamine, aspirin, and fish oil. The limp just became part of Penny, our phenomenal swimmer, a physical force who sometimes staggered. We almost accepted it.

Then one of her back legs stiffened. She elevated it, her toenails pitifully scraping the floor, or she placed both hind paws down as a single unit. She stared up at couches and our bed until we lifted her. She considered stairs and then decided against them. At only three years old, she was geriatric.

Arthritis was the most likely culprit. It often occurs in Labradors as a result of hip dysplasia, and symptoms can present as early as one year old.

I was nine months pregnant and, up until that moment, hadn't cried at sentimental commercials or baby sneakers balanced in my palm, but the idea of Penny cut down so early, denied the bliss of unencumbered movement, made my eyes sting.

Penny coiled on the couch beside me. I stuck my nose and fingers into the fur of her neck and my tears dampened her scruff. My protruding belly pushed against her backside, the pressure potentially paining her. Her hound eyes opened and shifted back to watch me, but she didn't resist.

At first glance, this natural progression of physical bodies appears to be deterioration, but a closer inspection reveals something more complicated. Humans are in constant flux (dogs too, apparently). We mature, and we acclimate. While we might lose dexterity and elasticity, we gain in other areas: sometimes wisdom, sometimes compassion, sometimes a crusty layered love, and sometimes, in our reinvention, we discover entirely novel talents. Where our waters hit a dam, they redirect.

We write "never change" in high school yearbooks, but that's because teenagers are dummies. Maybe that's too cruel. They're sentimental dummies. We do change. We must. And anyway, who wants to remain the narcissistic, melodramatic, reckless person they were at eighteen, even if it means eating an entire pizza pie without gaining weight, playing ice hockey at midnight, or propelling yourself into the air? We modify. We transfigure. We degrade in some ways but then we innovate and metamorphose. We are resilient.

Greg may not be game to backflip, but the essence of himself that seeks to push his body to its limit has found another way. He's started to run, and not the two-mile pedestrian jaunts I casually set out on, moving more vertically than horizontally, but ten-mile expeditions that take him through various neighborhoods of Boston before dumping him back on his doorstep, drenched and drained, but accomplished. His enduring spirit has adjusted his course.

Similarly, my dad has found fresh purpose in Rowen's care, and pleasure in his company. His eyes taper and his expression creases in ways I've never seen before, or at least in ways I don't remember and so appear new to me. Those fine crinkles are folded by time, but also by joy. My father still hurts, but he has reason to push through the pain, and comes out the other side reshaped into Grandpa. The photo of him as a young hockey player is still slipped into his mirror, but it's now surrounded by many more images of his grandson. What he's lost is outnumbered.

Then there's sweet Penny, who once shirked from children, who jumped off our bed and slept in the living room the night Rowen came home. She sniffs his head, or offers him a drive-by lick. Her heart is stretching to accommodate him, but her body will deteriorate before it improves.

When Rowen is six months old, tendons in both of Penny's knees will snap, weeks apart. She'll have double surgery, and for weeks we'll use a towel to harness her belly while she staggers on front legs. It'll take a full year, but she'll ease back into her previous activities, stiffer and with more reserve, but fueled by all the appreciation and whimsy of her youth. By then she'll have an eighteen-month boy bounding after her, who hugs and kisses her throughout the day, and whom she paws to on the couch so she can rest her head on his knee—even if it is only because he's streaked with peanut butter.

I too am in the outward process of decay, but internally, I am mercurial. The rooms of my heart are shifting and expanding. My brain is firing new synapses. The more I practice patience and tenderness, the less it feels like practice. I am loving deeper, and more unconsciously. I can almost see her now, the mother I am becoming.

In bed beside me, Rowen shudders in his sleep and pouts, and his rosy cheeks bulge. I press my lips against his small forehead and linger at that magnificent hairline. He smells like sweat, Greek yogurt, and something brand new.

This is as untouched as he will ever be. His precious newness—practically factory sealed—is expiring as we breathe together in the haze of morning, but will develop into vivacity and grace. His neck will strengthen until he can hold his head, his bones will lengthen, his feet will elongate. His skin, which now feels so plush, will cut, scrape, and burn. He'll totter, sprint, stumble, and bruise. He'll toughen. He'll throw, and he'll catch. He'll lift, leap, and dance. Then, though it seems impossible now, he will pay the cost of aging, just like the rest of us. His heels will crack. His bones will spur. His hair will thin. His spine will arch.

We don't know how he'll bud into a boy, blossom into a man, or in what ways he will use his physical self for expression, but we can hope that he will make the most of every movement; that, by the time he is a father, uncle, grandfather, when his joints, bones, and muscles aren't what they used to be, that he'll take comfort knowing they were put to good use, even if for too short a time; that they served others and demonstrated love; that they composed a vessel for a well-lived life; that his body was a celebration; and that when he grows weary, which only the lucky get to do, that he won't grieve what he's lost; that he'll appreciate the ways in which his evolution will urge him to recreate, and he'll rejoice in all the new parts of himself he uncovers; that he'll persevere, adapt, and find fresh utility in his new shape. That he will continue to live, and live well.

The Nest

When Rowen is four months old, a robin builds her nest on the windowsill outside our second-floor bathroom. It begins as a tuft of debris I think was blown onto the ledge by happenstance, but after enough furtive deliveries from its determined maker, I understand. The nest rises from the brick and shapes into a well-formed bowl spun from mud, grass, and sticks.

When the robin nests, her body absorbs her neck into a feathered teapot. Her back is colored like bark for camouflage, and she wears a swatch of marmalade on her breast for style. Her eyes are beady, almost accusatory, as she spots me spying from the other side of the glass. I don't dart out of the way in time, and she flits off.

Although I'm intrigued, I resist snooping on her. She's already put so much effort into her home; I don't want her to think she has to relocate. Mothering is hard enough. I know. For the past four months, outings don't seem worth the hassle of packing up, so I'll find it's Wednesday and I haven't changed from sweatpants since Sunday. I don't even know the weather; is it still spring? I wonder what everyone else is up to while I answer the call of my baby, putting aside whatever I was doing to lift my shirt and unfurl a swollen breast every two hours. They say newborns feed less frequently as they grow. Talk is cheap.

The monotony of baby-care is sometimes meditative, the tasks coming one after another in a sweet communion. Sometimes it's banal—another burping? another feeding? And sometimes restlessness is an itch inside my skin. While Rowen is physically attached to me, I find myself longing for a different sort of companionship, one of want rather than need, and personal connection rather than circumstance.

It's true that my attachment to Rowen is growing more robust by the day, alongside his personality. He grins at his music box, the artwork over his changing table, Neil Diamond's "Forever in Blue Jeans," *The Little Yellow Bee* book, and when we call him a "cool dude." I howl like wolf, and he stares at my mouth, kicks his legs, and yips back.

But I don't yet know how to operate as a mother inside my old life, with my former community and connections, nor have I found footing in this new one. I wonder if this is what it feels like when people spend enough years in a different land that all their languages become accented, the new one *and* their native tongue. I am a woman without a country.

I tote Rowen along to a new moms group, and slip off my shoes and join the circle of glassy-eyed women sitting cross-legged on colorful foam mats, their babies positioned before them like upside-down turtles. They share grievances about sleep and sore nipples and roll their eyes good-naturedly, but it seems like we are stiff actors reading scripts, not actually revealing anything true about ourselves. Or maybe it's just me. I smile along and nod when I should, but I'm playing a part, keeping my walls up so I am comfortably distanced. If this is a tribe, I'm just an observer, not a member. When I clip Rowen back into his car seat, I whisper, "I think it's just you and me, kid."

At least with the arrival of our feathered friend on the window ledge, I can study the easy proficiency of a new mother without having to pretend I have that quality myself.

To avoid adding a giant invader to the robin's list of burdens, I watch in stealth mode, approaching the window the way I sometimes tiptoe to the crib when the baby is too quiet and I want to make sure he is still breathing. One afternoon, I spy a drop of baby blue, like a single mini Cadbury egg, left in her twiggy dish.

I don't know if reproduction is a painful process for birds, but since there isn't an egg-size hole in her butt, I can guess. But the robin doesn't make a spectacle of birthing. She lays her eggs quietly and in private. One by one they appear, day after day, until there are four.

I sometimes spot another robin standing guard on the power line suspended over our street. He is twenty feet away but still in view of his nest, because robin parenting is a two-bird gig. Females are the primary nest builders and perform the majority of the feeding, but the males protect the nest from afar, and if a dad bird is killed, the mama might just abandon her young and start anew elsewhere, knowing it would be almost impossible to provide on her own.

Phil is more involved than the sentinel on the wires. He diapers, dresses, burps, and bounces. He's the only one to trim the baby's nails, what we call visiting Papa's Nail Salon. He swaddles using an ordinary sheet, while I require the Velcro handicaps. He woke for the feedings to keep me company and fluff the pillows until he returned to work and I assured him I'd prefer he sleep at night rather than in class, or worse, on his ride to school. He contributes as equal care as a work schedule allows, but since he simply doesn't have the anatomy, I am the primary feeder. Still, by ten weeks I'd pumped enough to accumulate stores of milk, so Phil began to bottle-feed a morning meal. With an extra four-hour block of sleep, people began to sound to me less like the adults from Charlie Brown.

While everyone else continues with the humdrum of their work lives, I stay home. The old me would have been talking to students, faculty members, and friends, asking questions and cataloguing answers, because learning is my primary love language. In lieu of that, I get to know Rowen, my flowering love, and I learn all I can about robins. (It's nice to get to know your neighbors.)

After she has laid her full clutch, the mama robin takes residence in her finely crafted dwelling, leaving only to hunt, and never for more than five minutes. Since feathers are too self-insulating, a section of the mama's tummy balds to create a brood patch; she parts her outer feathers and presses her bare belly against the eggs to share her body heat. When she's incubating, I miss the sight of the stunning, almost tropical-looking eggs, so unlike their drab mama, but I'm glad to know the eggs are keeping warm. It's May, and nights are still chilly. Besides, bedecked in my milk-stained hoodie and maternity stretch pants, I'm not one to judge outward appearances.

The robin looks content and self-assured in her perch. She knows where she's meant to be and what she's meant to do. She's pursuing her purpose, following built-in instincts while, on the other side of the wall, I'm there too, balanced on the toilet like a gal pal in the next bathroom stall, begging for the secret ingredient.

The eggs could take two weeks to hatch. The timing is perfect, really, because my family is going on vacation and will return in plenty of time for the first crack.

Phil and I usually use the summer months for a grand adventure, but since parenting is grand enough, we are plopping down at a riverfront house only a couple hours north. There won't be a town for twenty-five minutes, and no neighbors to be bothered by nighttime cries. The closest food source will be a woman who sells pie out of her kitchen.

This trip marks a milestone of some kind. Veteran parents say the first three months are the hardest. Exhaustion and frustration can drive parents to desperation—sometimes clinical insanity.

My baby had all the dreamy hallmarks of a newborn—sweet breath, soft skin, and fat feet I couldn't resist squeezing. If God gives you only what you can handle, He didn't think much of me because He gave me the most agreeable baby in his workshop. (I may be confusing God with Santa Claus.) But Rowen also had erratic sleep patterns, poop that seeped through his onesie and onto my leg, an unquenchable hunger, and, worst of all, no means to appreciate my efforts. In fact, he still only regularly smiles for Phil, even when I perform like a slapstick comedian, crashing into doors and contorting my features. I aspired to be an author for over a decade and didn't consider myself to be someone in need of recognition, but being expected to dote on and love someone who showed no signs of loving me back was like writing with disappearing ink. At Rowen's first smile, though, the letters I'd scrawled began to materialize.

My body, too, is on the mend. I am still spilling blood, milk, and salt, and my pulverized pelvis regularly complains, but the empty husk of my stomach is tucking itself into the pants of my torso, and the linea nigra is reabsorbing. I am beginning to look like someone I recognize.

To honor our progress, at four months, Phil and I land on a river in Maine as wearied travelers newly arrived, our baby and dog in tow.

My family indulges in baked berries, watches the dog swim, and feeds, feeds, feeds. I'm struck by how like a hatchling my dear one is, his neck made wobbly by the weight of his head, his round searchlight eyes, the wrinkle of fat shrinking on his wrist, his sweet coos and babble.

I happily calendar the progress the birds are making in our absence. Upon our return, there will still be another week before a chick uses its egg tooth as a hatchet to break through its shell. Since there are four eggs, this struggle will span half a week. They'll spill out as bony sacks of pink skin, eyes sealed closed. At any sign of their mama, presumably returning with food, they'll transform into giant open upturned beaks. During daylight hours, the robin parents will experience a new frenzy. The hatchlings will need to eat every half hour, and since their nutrition doesn't come from a breast, they will have to source the food, hunting for insects, fruit, and worms nonstop. No recreational soaring. No bird friends. No Tweeter. (Sorry.) This is their new normal.

By the trip's end, I don't want to leave Maine, where we are cocooned from trying to accommodate naps, diaper changes, and nursing into other agendas, simply operating by our own rhythms and that of the tidal river, where I don't even try to fit the new me into my old life. But I oddly do look forward to returning to the nest in time for the proud, practiced mama to meet her hatchlings. I want to share in her joy and know-how.

Once home, I go straight to the window, but the nest is gone.

I tear down the stairs and out the front door, where I find what by then I already expect. The sculpted nest has reverted to the detritus of its parts—clumps of dirt, hay, and sprigs plucked from our neighborhood now speckled with shards of baby blue.

It must have been the cat who prowls, taunts my dog, and startles drivers. If not him, then a bullying blue jay. It doesn't matter who it was. What's done is done. When I see the mess, I groan.

I pity the robin who worked so hard and lost so much. She was a natural. She got motherhood right from the start. What a shame to squander those instincts. She is a parent without her hatchlings while, now returned to the backdrop of my former life, I am a woman in the dark, clutching my child in one hand and groping the wall with the other.

Over the next few days, I unconsciously check the window whenever I use the bathroom, and experience a small letdown of sadness at the sight of the empty ledge.

Rowen slept across the hall from us in Maine because the lighting in the master bedroom was too bright. We figure this is as good a time as any to move him to his nursery. Though we'd grown accustomed to this setup over our getaway, it's almost a brand-new adjustment back home. Without him directly beside me, kicking, mewling, and even snoring, I feel as if I finally have room to take a full breath, but also like part of my body has been removed and placed on the other side of the wall.

I'm woken by phantom Rowen sounds all night. I'm sure he's crying, but when I go to him, he's peaceful in his crib. I don't mind the interruption so much as worry I'll eventually convince myself all cries are imaginary, and won't go to him when he needs me. Or worse, it won't occur to me when he's gone too long without making any sounds at all.

I shiver to wonder how that robin coped the night her nest was destroyed. Where did she wait out the darkness, the feeling of four lumps beneath her suddenly, irrevocably, gone?

The experience of motherhood is so varied, but that is, perhaps, one universal—the dread of the worst possibility: a nest no longer intact. I fret that I'm not doing this right, but what's infinitely worse, unbearable to ponder, is the idea of not getting to do it anymore at all, having my title, so new it sits rigidly around my shoulders, ripped from me, but only externally. Internally, the coding has already been made permanent. At a mother's death, the foreign cells of her children can be found floating in her blood and bones, whether they hatched or not.

The unthinkable fear I carry with me like a pit is proof of my induction into the association of new mothers. I don't have to build my resume and apply for entry, I haven't been accidentally recruited, nor am I weighing down the team. I can grant myself permission to own this identity, and to look to other parents as my peers. If motherhood doesn't feel like it looks, that's because it isn't one size fits all, except in this particular way: I've joined the ranks of the worried.

Every other concern is trivial when held up against the ultimate terribleness, so I shouldn't quibble over how I might have behaved or how I hope I will feel tomorrow. Rather, I should accept and appreciate things as they are, because seconds slipped-by are gone for good. I'll never have another spring with Rowen as he is now. By next year he'll be walking, so I must cradle him while I can, inhale him while I can, and pull him close inside the stillness of our shared simple pleasures: shadows shifting across the ceiling, the sharp green of a newly sprouted leaf, a smile passed from baby to mother, a woman pushing a stroller outside our window, and—what's this?—the hopeful lilt of a bird's song.

Letter to Women Who Fear Childbirth

To my dear pot roast-footed insomniacs, the back-aching, full-bladdered, kangaroo-bellied time bombs:

People dread public speaking, waking for an early flight, and Mondays. You are allowed to dread being carved out from the inside.

It's normal to be scared of childbirth. It has to be. Anyone who claims otherwise is a big fat liar. I have no evidence to back that up, but it feels true enough that I might post it on a Wikipedia entry. Then it'll definitely be true.

Women confront the stuff of folklore, come out the other side, and return uncelebrated to their regular lives—inputting data, sipping coffee, composing emails—while their siege recedes into private legend. There should be parades in their honor. Statues erected. National holidays. Medals pinned to pashminas and free lattes for life. Instead, their harrowing act is commemorated annually by lighting candles . . . for someone else.

Giving birth is a formidable undertaking. Good thing you are formidable.

All your life you've been told to smile, be nice, and behave like a lady. But behaving like a lady doesn't mean submission, graciousness, or accommodations. It is having mythic ability. It is challenging anguish with your battle-ax. It's been this way for as long as there has been human life.

Your body has been preparing you. It knows what to do. Your waters will break through their levee. Your bones will make way and your muscles will press down. You will tremble, shudder, and quake, but you will soften, and you will open.

It's going to suck. So bad. You will cry out. You will hurl everything you have into the black. (If you want anesthesia, by God, take it, woman.) You'll beg for it to end, and it will, it will. Like everything, it will end.

When it does, and the dust settles, and the sun evaporates the fog, your feet will shrink, your bladder will reclaim its space, and your old clothes will begin to fit again. There's all that to look forward to, as well as a new person to learn. It might take a beat, but you are going to adore that little bugger, and not just because he adores you (though that helps). At the sight of one another, you will light up as two old friends reuniting, even when you've only just gone to the bathroom.

Post-delivery, you might feel traumatized. Why shouldn't you? You've been through something serious. Almost every other mother has been through it too. They thrummed their war drums through contractions. They pushed like they were pooping until they finally delivered life from their bodies. It's okay to share your hurt. They'll hear you, girl. They'll see you. (While you're at it, tell the men too— preferably while they're eating.)

If nothing else, I hear you. I see you.

Alena

PS. By the way, it's acceptable to wear your maternity jeans until kindergarten drop-off day. You deserve the panels. You've earned *the panels.*

PART VII

Beyond

Mothering in the Time of Coronavirus

April 2020

THE LAND OF THE FREE IS HOME BEING BRAVE.

My body wants to sleep and wake up when this is all over, to skip ahead and look back at 2020 with the clear vision of its name. I want to be told how it turned out with the pacing and drama of not having lived it: *The scientists were brilliant and the medical workers were valiant and the people were vigilant and when they came together again they were stronger and more appreciative and loved better than ever.*

But Rowen is fourteen months old. His little piston arms pump as he sprints around the house. My instinct is to hibernate, but his consciousness is coming alive more each day. Gears turn behind his eyes as he furrows his brow and assembles small epiphanies: *There's the tree that housed all those chirping sparrows yesterday, so where are they today? There used to be a flower in a vase on the table for me to sniff. Where did it go?* Every new movement—climb onto the couch, crawl up the stairs, bend knees and jump!—is a feat. Every new word is a stone turned to reveal a tiny ecosystem.

The people who love him—oh so fiercely, oh so desperately—have to keep their distance and miss this. I can't. I won't. I force my eyes open and pay attention to every object he points to, every word he repeats and pats into his memory.

Still, I feel like a battery drained to, what? Seventy percent? Forty? Am I sick, or is this exhaustion because I had to tell my parents they couldn't visit their grandson?

My son peers into our guest room. "Nonna?"

"No, Baby. Nonna isn't here."

My friends place bets on when we can have a drink in a bar again. Loser buys. No one guesses beyond July 1—three months away. We can't bear to.

I have fifteen family members in New York City, the pandemic epicenter of the world. What's the mortality percentage of that?

Rowen doesn't wonder such things. He presses the button on his music box and stomps along to "Rockin' Robin." He smiles with a little mountain range of teeth.

"Papa?" he asks.

"Yes, Baby. Papa is downstairs. He's working at home now."

During my work shift, I stare at the laptop and my words stare back, self-conscious and inert. They are flatter than the curve. It's as if they know they don't matter.

My son pounds on my bedroom door. "Sorry, dude. Mimi is working," Phil says from the other side, but I let Rowen in, relieved to be interrupted. He sticks a flower in my face and wrinkles his own nose, prompting me. The flower is artificial. I smell anyway.

"So pretty, Baby. Thank you for that sniff."

Every day, new articles are published about the coronavirus. It's impossible to read them all, but I try. What else is there to do? I learn there will likely be outbreaks after this one. The second wave of the Spanish flu was worse than the first. Even if a vaccine is developed, the virus could mutate enough to be invulnerable to it. Those who have been sick may be sick again.

Baby gazes out the window, his eyes so blue and bright. He isn't tired of his surroundings. He doesn't feel bound up or caged. He is opening, discovering. There are infinite possibilities just inside the confines of our house, countless objects to inspect, taste, or throw. Behind every cabinet door is a galaxy of steel, fabric, or plastic. Then there's the world on the other side of the window, also wondrous and ever-changing, but not necessarily more so, and it's enough that we get to gaze at it from afar. His forehead falls against mine.

"Caaah."

"Yes, Baby. That car is driving so fast. Where do you think it's going?"

We walk our dog three times a day to get a change of scenery. When we pass someone on the sidewalk, we hold our breath. Others emerge from their houses and squint against the sunshine. When their eyes adjust, they might be smiling at us, but it looks a lot like sadness. We are wearing masks, so I wave in a way that I hope seems bright and friendly.

"Bahhbahh."

"Yes, Baby. Waving is a nice thing to do, isn't it?"

Once, when we are carrying Rowen around the block, he points to our neighbor's granddaughter. "Delia, Delia." He doesn't lunge for her, as he did weeks ago. He should be tottering on playgrounds, attending library music hours, and trading blocks and spit with other kids, but instead he's learning to keep his distance. This virus is altering us, whether it's in our cells our not.

"Go on," I say. "Show Delia your best monkey face."

We check in on each other the only way we can: we text, we call, we Zoom. My brother, Ryan, says he got out of bed at one in the afternoon, showered, cried, and went back to bed. My brother, Greg, lives alone. How can someone be alone through this?

"How are you?" I ask.

"Existing," Greg says.

We aren't sick, but we aren't well.

Baby needs to eat. At least that's something to do.

"Nanana," he says.

"Sorry, Baby. We're out of bananas. I'll get more on our next supply run."

He waves at me from his highchair. I'm sitting directly in front of him, but I must have seemed far away. He brings me back.

"Hello, Baby."

He offers me one of his puffs, and delights when I nibble it from his dimpled hands. Feeding us brings him joy.

We are down to canned vegetables and watered-down half-and-half for Rowen's bottle, so I go shopping. They restrict the number of people allowed inside, so fifteen shoppers wait outside in a staggered line. A store employee stands at the entrance and yells, "Six feet apart. Starbucks is closed. Six feet apart."

I'm looking at two packages of chicken breasts in an otherwise empty case. The entire section is refrigerated and illuminated for eight measly chicken breasts. From behind a hand-sewn mask, a woman says, "They have meat. Isn't it wonderful?"

There is one jug of milk and its sell-by date is today. Or yesterday. Or tomorrow. I feel lucky to have gotten anything and guilty for taking the last one, but Rowen has to drink. I'll separate the milk into small containers and freeze them so it'll keep longer, the way my mother does because she can't get through a gallon on her own and buying quarts is more expensive. It's a practice I said I'd never do. Now is never.

As I climb into the car, I keep track of everything I touch and retrace my steps with an alcohol wipe: keys, purse, door handle. Then I rip off my mask and take my first unrestricted breath in forty minutes.

When I get home, my heart is racing from the expedition, and I expect a hero's welcome. I am Hunter and Gatherer. I am agitated. I am exhausted. I am getting a migraine. My husband disinfects the cereal boxes. They say we don't have to, but they used to tell us not to wear masks, and now there are bandana tutorials all over social media and a mandatory mask order in town.

My head still throbs, but Rowen needs a new diaper. He smiles at me from the changing table. "Stinkay."

"Yes, Baby. It is."

His bowel movement is abnormal. He doesn't feel warm, but I check for fever anyway.

The next week, I go for a bike ride. It's hardly an innovative idea.

There are more bikers out than ever before. You cover more distance biking than jogging, and we want to see as much as possible before returning to our own four walls. Or maybe it's because biking is faster, and we hope, on wheels, the virus won't catch us.

It's Easter Sunday and church parking lots are empty. New York City averaged seven hundred deaths a day this week. I wonder if the family of the deceased and the medical workers who fought so hard to keep them alive are envious of Mary and the disciples. Jesus laid down his life but got to rise again.

The beach is closed. Concrete barriers block the parking lot, the entrance is cordoned off with yellow caution tape, and a policeman patrols. A flashing traffic sign reads *Covid-19 Outbreak. No parking, stopping, or standing.* A line of cars crawls up the hill and circles the roundabout to catch a glimpse of the most beautiful place we have.

I glide around the loop for my dose. Maybe I linger too long. A man shouts at me from his car, "It's spiritual, isn't it?"

I'd normally laugh at such a granola notion, but it is, it is. I'm not supposed to, but the sand stretches like a yawn and the waves lap gently and the coast is rugged and untouched, so I take another turn.

A few miles from my house, I pull my bike to the side of the road to jot a note on my phone.

"Are you all right?" a walker yells from across the street.

I assure her yes, but I think, *If I wasn't, how could she help? What could she do?*

Later, a fellow biker lifts a face shield to wipe tears from her eyes. It's sixty degrees and sunny, the first real day of spring. She's biking with an acrylic face shield and crying. But how can I help? What can I do?

I arrive home sweaty and red-faced, but Rowen throws his arms around my knees, and although this is the place I've been for four weeks straight, I'm happy to be back. I tickle his neck and he laughs like wind chimes. We play in the backyard. We are fortunate to have our own bit of green space when playgrounds, parks, trails, and beaches are off-limits. It's a type of currency, wealth of the new world, like toilet paper and antibodies.

Rowen snaps off a piece of grass and presses it against his nose. We are so fragile. We are so worried. He extends it to me, but just as I lean in to mime a sniff, he drops the blade and points to the sky. A seagull soars overhead. I don't remember seagulls coming inland this far, but maybe it's the kind of scenery I'm noticing only when my son brings it to my attention. Or maybe the absence of people is changing the natural order of things, and when we finally emerge from our houses, it will be to an altered landscape. My son's finger follows the shadow as it glides with grace, seemingly weightless.

"Biihhrd."

Rowen's expression is full of wonder. That ordinary sighting, a seagull's modest wingspan—it's enough for him. His childlike reverence is a sort of wisdom, and my own personal miracle. It's enough. It's essential. He's so much.

"Yes, Baby. Isn't that something?"

A Reflection on the First Two Years

PHIL ONCE TOLD ME THAT HE USED TO LOVE IN BLACK AND WHITE, AND only when he met me did he start loving in color. (Heartthrob alert.) That's a fair assessment of how my relationship with Rowen began. I was rolled from the delivery room into a monochromatic world. Everything, even what I'd before observed in a spectrum of color, was suddenly muted by stress, foreign terrain, chemical imbalance, physical trauma, and exhaustion. The saturation increased as Rowen crinkled his nose, as he opened his mouth for applesauce as if for an aria, and as his laughter effervesced into neon bubbles around our heads, until I was witnessing with more intensity and contrast than ever before. I emerged from postpartum depression the way I emerged from morning sickness—a slow, almost imperceptible, return to myself. I wanted the scenery to burst into Technicolor from the start, as Dorothy entering Oz, the same way we wish we could clear old romances from our histories, but perhaps it is only when we hold former dullness against our current lives that we appreciate its vibrancy.

Over the past two years—or, to omit the fever dream of the fourth trimester, twenty-one months—bursts of light have been plentiful and kaleidoscopic: when Rowen's chubby legs launched him to his feet for the first time, and he turned to me with a flower of pride opening behind his expression; when he lowered his face into his bathwater—cautiously, so cautiously—and turned to me to share in the amusement of his wet nose and mouth; when he followed the same route around the house like a cop on his beat, pausing only at anomalies, a leaf brought in on the sole of a shoe, for instance, which he plunked down to examine, turning it over in his right hand and then his left; when his vocalizations ranged from guttural Russian to nasal Portuguese, as if he were born with all languages at once; when we played hide-and-seek and he left his spot to help us look for him; the night we realized he'd memorized his favorite book; his first attempt down the cascade of "L, M, N, O, P"; when he raised his arm in his stroller and said, "Holdy hand, Mimi?" and I laced my fingers through his so that, once again, we were connected as if by an umbilical cord, with him contained before me; when, after a night away, he beheld our house as if it were snowing inside, so transfixed was he to see his blocks, his dog, and his couch, logging all his belongings as if to say, "It's still here. It's all still here."

These delights helped me rise from the ashes, but melancholy left streaks of char behind. The disturbance of not recognizing newborn Rowen has delayed me from cutting his hair, to prevent a reoccurrence. Bangs maintenance was necessary when he started walking into walls, so I trimmed them when he was nine months old, snipping slowly, inspecting his face for transformation. To my immense relief, fine hairs clung to the plastic of his highchair, but below his freshly shorn edges, jagged from my split focus, was my baby, looking more mature, but still mine. The rest of his mane remains untouched, growing wilder by the day. At two years old, he looks like a sun-kissed Kevin Sorbo Hercules, his locks bouncing with sporadic corkscrew curls. It's glorious, and I intend to preserve and honor it like a shrine.

My brain didn't release love hormones automatically. How unfair for my sweet baby. He deserved better than that. But he was patient, and he was tenacious. By the very act of existing in the world, he made his way back through my body and manually reprogrammed my wiring until my glands were pumping out the good stuff and we were swimming in chemical love. He did that.

I don't know what would have accelerated the process and, by proxy, the bond with my son. Maybe despondency was something I had to wade through—the cost of assembling a new human. Maybe spawning Rowen's joy meant draining some from me, and it took time to replenish my stock. Maybe our vision had to develop in synchrony, since his also began as a blurry spectrum of gray. I wonder if it'll feel more natural next time around, with mothering circuits prewired, but maybe not. Maybe each child is someone you learn anew.

There will always be something special and intrepid about this first experience. Rowen was the explorer who braved this course with me. I was a co-trailblazer, or maybe the alpaca. Either way, we entered this unknown territory together. Just as I birthed him into the world, he birthed me into an altered version of myself. We made one another. Neither was fast or painless. Each required gestation, patience, nurturing, and forgiveness. He expanded my ribs and enriched my brain.

Now I wear an R pendant around my neck. I anticipate the autonomy bedtime provides only to spend that freedom watching videos of him. When Rowen is hollering with the full range of his lungs, it doesn't matter if Phil has comforted him to stillness. His despair reverberates in my cells, as if the DNA he left behind is radiating. I am not right until I hold him and bury my nose in the places his smell is most concentrated—the crook of his neck, his palms, his mouth—sniffing as if to inhale him back into myself.

Since women are born with all of their eggs already stored in their ovaries, half of what would become Rowen was born with me, and I carried that part of him to summer camps and choir practice, into reading nooks and high school keggers, off to college and job interviews, until Phil completed the formula and I delivered that extension of myself, for the first time in thirty-two years, out of my body. Now all I have is what he left behind. I hope those cells make their way into my heart and brain.

* * * * *

As a parent of a toddler, my limbs have been put to use tossing, dancing, crawling, clomping, clapping, lifting my toes to my nose, widening my mouth until my lips strain, sticking my tongue out, and baring teeth.

Rowen and I bellow cheek to cheek, listening to one other's volume and tone, mimicking or departing from our partner, only to return to a collective note. It isn't biking through Hyde Park or hiking fjords. It isn't sipping cabernet in Napa or kayaking the Amalfi Coast water caves. But it is a capability we have at our disposal anytime we feel the urge, without the need for passports, investment, or reservations. We don't have to rush from one thing to the next. We can hunker down and enjoy the view inside our house (which is a handy pastime during a worldwide pandemic). We can be jubilant, furious, and loud. We can express ourselves and be heard. So, my God, we bellow.

We sing every day. Breakfast, naptime, bedtime, in the car, while cleaning up toys, on a walk. Nursery rhymes, Irish tunes, Disney favorites, Christmas carols, oldies, and radio hits. Solos, duets, and as a chorus. Rowen makes requests, and we sing. There are songs drifting from my untrained vocal cords so often the sound has eroded my self-consciousness. I launched into "Circle of Life" in front of the zoo's lion cage and didn't stop until my brother remarked, "You know there are other people here, right?"

The love of a child is without fear of rejection or vulnerability. It isn't self-conscious. It is pummeling. When Rowen sees me, his expression is a window thrown open. He bashes into me with his full force. He fills me up.

There's a new layer to all my experiences. Something pulses beneath them like a heart. He's altered my timbre. Sometimes I hear myself comfort him, and I sound so nurturing, foreign to my own ears, and wonder if being as round as the Chinese Buddha during pregnancy somehow infused me with zen.

Perhaps what's thrilled me most is Rowen's sense of humor. Timing can't be taught, and this kid's got it. At just the right moment, he'll announce, "Fart coming!" Sometimes, straddling my lap, nose to nose, he'll shoot me a certain look, and we'll tumble into a giggling bout the likes of which I haven't had since I was a girl awake with friends at two in the morning. He performs impersonations that topple me, and then he follows close behind, his small shoulders juddering, his smile shoving his cheeks to his ears. When one of us settles, the other surges, and we seesaw until we're breathless.

I think back to when I was desperate to know anything about the fetus zapping my strength and beauty. If I could have seen how this person would emerge like a shape lifting out of clay into a longhaired, joke-telling, outdoors boy who sniffs flowers and identifies birdcalls; an animal lover who stoops next to Penny and asks, "You okay, baby girl?"; a reader and charmer as distinct as those kids at the Queen concert; a sensitive friend, attentive enough to say, "Good job walking, Mimi,"; an exquisite creature, his muscles and tendons stretching like a well-tuned stringed instrument; I would have invited the tearing open of my body, anything to have him at last.

He's but a single brushstroke against the canvas of the universe, yet he's already learned that when you stumble upon something of value, you should clutch it as a stone in your hand. He practices this with literal stones, of course, but more meaningfully, he mulls memories, tasting them over and over again.

"Fox. Walk. Stroller. Street," he said at eighteen months old, pointing out the window.

"Yes, Baby. We saw a fox run across the street while we were walking in the stroller."

He nodded, wide eyed, still not believing our luck, only to recap the event ten minutes later. What would have at best amounted to a passing comment to Phil—"Hey, I saw a fox on my run"—developed into family legend. But wasn't it lucky, that wily streak of copper, with her black stockings hiked thigh high? Shouldn't I be awed?

Sometimes I find myself peering at Rowen as if through a porthole into a country I can't quite understand, because it is no longer my own. What prompted his fascination with the mailman? What gave him the idea that dogs want to sniff his armpit? Why does a kiss mollify his hurts? Why is he eating Penny's kibble . . . again? Why is he an absolute darling in one breath and completely unreasonable in the next, in turn revealing the best and worst in me?

My son invigorates and exasperates me in equal measure. There are the common aggravations of teething, gas, and sleep regressions, or swatting food into a Jackson Pollock I must scrape from the wall. There are more significant heartbreaks, like removing bottles from rotation and enduring pleas of "Baba" that are so mournful I wonder if I could just let him chug milk from rubber nipples until prom. But it's the temper tantrums that drag me into wells of despair.

I check the clock in the midst of feet-stomping, tears-leaping-from-ducts mornings, certain it must almost be tomorrow, and think, *My god. Only nine thirty?*

The most minor grievances—offering the blue spoon rather than the green spoon, or the green spoon rather than the blue spoon, or the wrong pizza slice—can rile him to absolute turbulence. He tilts his face toward the ceiling as if to beseech, "Why, God? Why?" with tears torrenting his face, and by then it doesn't matter how many blue spoons or green spoons or whole pizza pies I shove at his clenched fists, saying, "Here, just take it!" He is inconsolable. He's perceptive enough to know what he wants, but his smallness is a cage through which splendor dances out of reach. Sometimes his limitations aren't bothersome. Other times he grips the bars and roars.

Toddlers can't regulate their emotions, and their stress is compounded by powerlessness. I empathize with that on a theoretical level, but as he expresses his irrational opposition, my blood pressure rises. I can't reason with him, and I can't soothe him, so I am equally out of control. I feel just as he feels, only it's not acceptable for me to claw, bite, or throw my cup of milk. We are two toddlers in the throes of tempests, but I'm repressed.

When Rowen was sixteen months old, Phil and I took him to the beach. He was jubilant, snatching up pebbles and tossing them into the sea, squealing with delight. He pointed to seagulls and grinned as the frosty water sloshed his toes, and the sun was warm and sailboats floated on the horizon. It was true magic, which I tried to recreate on my own the following day. I slathered on sunscreen, wriggled him into a bathing suit, and packed his diaper bag with a towel, a change of clothes, snacks, and sand toys. (Okay, old Tupperware containers.)

I parked the car and hauled him and our stuff from the lot to the beach, arriving slick with sweat. As I lowered him to the sand, his eyes tapered and he wailed.

"But you love the beach. Remember the pebbles? You throw them in the water," I said eagerly, grabbing a handful. "And the seagulls? Hear them squawk? Or the waves. We can play in the waves." I placed him down. I picked him up. I ran around. I tossed him in the air. I carried him from one end of the beach to the other. He yowled like he was a vampire being fried by the sun. The thrill of the previous day was irrelevant. My distractions were useless. It didn't matter that we'd been locked down by a pandemic for months and this was a desperate breath of fresh air. His desires prevailed. He was ruling with a mighty fit.

"Home. Car. Bye-bye," he said, between sobs.

I stuffed our towel back in the diaper bag, hefted it over one shoulder, and scooped him with my other arm. He smelled of suntan lotion, whose clumsy application had been unnecessary. He'd ruined my day at the beach, and pleasure is worth something, no matter how small. Rage amassed inside me. I wanted to open a valve, and he was too young to understand what was on my mind, so I loosed it.

"Fine, we're going home," I said. "Fuck you."

I was aiming for catharsis, and it did indeed release some pressure, but I'll grapple with its ugliness for months, maybe the rest of my life, along with the too-familiar temper that sidles up beside me during his tantrums and wraps its arm around my shoulder. Usually I can shrug it off, but sometimes I can't, and it clings to me long enough that I adopt its stench, and it requires a degree of intention not to shake Rowen a little, or bend into his face and shout, "Drink from the damn sippy cup. It's not your bottle, but it's all the same milk!"

Occasionally, when Rowen's insolence is especially unrelenting, visions of violence sear across my imagination like a locomotive. I barely get a glimpse of their oily sheen before they roar by, but I see enough to shiver, and the scream of their whistles echoes in my ears.

I manage to internalize my frustration, but I wish it didn't rumble inside me in the first place. I wouldn't invite a serial killer to a dinner party even if he promised not to act on homological urges. It's still what he'll be thinking about, and who he is. Likewise, if I resist my impulses, it's still part of who I am, and still affects me, fossilizing my person inside and out. My lips thin. My body congeals. I remember my mother from when I was a kid, worn by responsibility, bemoaning, "I used to be a fun person." I can see myself being battered down to that lament, and I don't want "fun" to be a characteristic from my past. I want Rowen to know that part of me. But perhaps where there is immense love, there must also be its opposite, and for a mother to disparage herself for experiencing the inevitable foil to joy is as futile as begrudging day for yielding to night.

I'd like to believe the truly patient parent can't exist—like easy babies or tasty Swiss chard—except I live with one. Phil's levelheaded (dead inside) reaction after peeling a writhing, twenty-five-pound tear-stained toddler from the floor because he wasn't allowed to throw a glass jar down the stairs is sympathy. "He can't communicate his emotions," Phil might say. "I feel bad for him." So do I, but I also feel bad for us. We're the ones who live with an insane glass-hurling despot.

I'm ashamed by how I mismanage his meltdowns, especially since my equitable arrangement with Phil means I watch Rowen for only half the day. I often think, *I lost my patience, and we were together only four hours*, as if that block is my minimum obligation, so inside it I should perform at the height of my capacity. Since fathers aren't expected to take on so much, Phil views the same four-hour block as a certificate of achievement. If he wants to lie on the floor and close his eyes, he'll think, *It's fine. We are together four hours*. Phil's ahead in the father race, while I'm behind the mother starting line.

I question whether I capitalized every moment. Should I have watched him sleep rather than tiptoed out of his room to grade papers? Should I have lowered to the ground and raced cars rather than collapsing on the couch? I should pay close attention, and live inside these presents before they are part of my past.

It was only two years ago that this now-toddler wailed into a delivery room, purple and furious. His vision was blurred and his skeleton was cartilage. His skull was misshaped, his features swollen, and his belly button a wound. All the days that brought us here to his boyhood felt infinite in the moment and instant in retrospect. I fell asleep while he was warm dough on my chest, so small I cupped his backside with one palm, and woke to skinned knees and legs dangling down my hip. That's how quickly it changed. Now he eats Brussels sprouts, waves to the garbageman, and ricochets down playground slides. Inside my next breath he'll climb the steps of a school bus, turn the ignition of his first car, and drive away from our unit to create his own. I should savor every moment and then catch it by its tail as it slips by, because each second is a precious bit of him I can't get back. Why am I typing this sentence when I should be taking advantage of the finite time he wants to play with Mimi?

But how do you appreciate every moment when they are lined up one behind the other, so many in a row they narrow into the horizon? It's like trying to relish a heaping bowl of ice cream. After a while, your tongue grows numb, even to ambrosia.

At the same time, if I let myself think too much about how fast he is growing, and how soon this time will be over, my heart begins to pound.

* * * * *

I criticize my mothering performance, but I also see how I've been personally compromised. I used to be efficient, organized, and productive. I made to-do lists. I organized our pantry. I optimized our budget, shopped for deals, and ordered thoughtful birthday gifts. I used stillness to foster more order. Now there's no stillness. I can't bother with price comparisons or birthday gift shopping, so I send cash. I don't vacuum under the couch, dust the picture frames, or scrub mineral deposits from around the bathtub drain. Did I plant a garden this season? That's hilarious. We would have thrown ourselves a small party for mowing the lawn, but we didn't have time.

Our house is a wreck because Rowen doesn't play with toys so much as rearrange our closets, and we've grown weary of roping them shut (with literal slipknots of Phil's creation, of course), or distracting Rowen with one of the many puzzles, paint sets, or interactive toddler games that go unused. Instead, we've conceded, storing canisters of oats on the top shelf of the pantry so they don't spill. We are remodeled by a toddler's whims, and because of that surrender, the sunscreen is under the couch cushions, the remote control is in the junk drawer, and the peanut butter has been swapped with the toothpaste. Social media casts parenting under the idealized filter of an autumn photo shoot, every turned leaf in just the right place, but the truth is it's messy and unrefined. It shines a light on your humanity, your tender places as well as your jagged edges. When I reach for a fork but discover paraphernalia of an adjacent f-word, I appreciate it as an apt summary of parenting: the lube is with the silverware.

• • • • •

I would fight with my teeth to secure what Rowen deserves and establish what's best for him, but often I just don't know what that is. Should I transfer him from my lap, where he eats with prayerful earnestness, to his highchair? Should we enforce structure on the rest of mealtimes, or continue his grazing habit because it celebrates *joie de vivre*? Should we revoke the pacifier, or would it be too traumatizing when he can't understand its disappearance? Should we protect his naptime or practice adaptability? Does drawing hard lines provoke gratuitous unpleasantness in an already gratuitously unpleasant world?

It's pandemic time, so other parents are stowed away in their houses, but when they venture out, I look to them for guidance. Rowen ambles onto playground equipment and I say, "Wait, dude, I have to come with you," but when another mother allows her toddler the independence, I adjust, saying, "Oh, actually, go ahead, I guess."

I may not be a practiced parent, or even altogether confident, but as I shift Rowen from one hip to the other, tuck his hair behind his ear, graze my finger along a rash, and kiss his scraped palm better, I'm learning, lengthening, and acquiring a certain fluidity and grace. I'm beginning to realize that I'm good enough. Sometimes I don't rise to the occasion as I wish, but more often than not, I do. Rowen runs to me, I scoop him up, and he fits perfectly into my side. We nuzzle, tickle, talk, and laugh—we love—and in those moments, I feel that I've arrived.

My evolution isn't nearly over. I'll continue to bend, elongate, dig deeper, toughen, and soften. It happened to my own mother. In photographs from when we were babies, she glows as if there's a lamp beneath her skin, or as if she'd just flung open a door to a cool, floral-laced breeze. That's what loving young children did for her. The mother I remember knew what she was doing—she was proficient, but aggravated by her overextension. The mother in the photograph, however, holding the amorphous cherub by the armpits, was unsure of her abilities, but exuberant.

By the time Rowen's memories establish staying power, I'll have changed in much the same way. He might look back at photographs of me as a young mother—when his legs bestrode my waist, we stared into each other's eyes, our foreheads kissed, and we laughed at a private joke—and he'll recognize the woman carrying him, but the version he'll know will be seasoned. Wise, but wizened. The luminous person in the image, her green youthfulness and apologetic uncertainty, will make her a sweet stranger.

He won't remember me as I am now, or the dearness of our time together when he was small: how we depend upon one another for company and comfort; how we share every meal, me often cutting his food with my teeth to make it safe; how I bathe him, sometimes climbing into the tub myself; how we hold hands when we walk; how I am acquainted with the intricacies of his every day—who he sees, how he plays, his moods; how I'm versed in what disturbs and fascinates him; how I'm fluent in his particular and sometimes peculiar language—"mama" for oatmeal, "ah-ah" for vacuum, and "big boy" for chair; how we cling to one another as we rock in the chair beside his crib; how we nest our bodies on a bed piled with books and stuffed animals; and how he calls for me each morning when he wakes. To realize he won't remember the fierce intimacy of these years is to know your best friend will one day forget you.

He'll likely reflect on his childhood the way I do mine, through the survival mechanism that latches onto memories of stress, retaining unpleasantness so as to avoid it in the future. Grownup Rowen will love me, but he'll also bear in mind my flaws, my mistakes, as a means of protection, so he won't commit them himself, while I'll do the opposite, for my own preservation.

By then my veins will have surfaced as ropes beneath papery skin, the loose skin of my stomach will sag, my hair will be silver and coarse, and my bare breasts won't look appealing even when I raise my arms over my head. The strength and vitality of my physical body will be mostly behind me, as will much of my joy.

I'll fawn over Rowen's childhood, gripping my fondness the same way his one-year-old self gripped stones, romanticizing his youth into an ideal, because our shared history will be what sustains me as I drift toward my own personal sunset, carrying bits of him with me in my bones. All the tantrums, worries, uncertainties, doubts, melancholy, and tears will be rubbed smooth by retrospect, while the raptures will stand in my rearview mirror as pronounced and resplendent as a mountain range. I'll dwell in the past, remembering Rowen as he stood vigil with Penny during thunderstorms, or how his small off-key singing was so elated and barefaced, his eyebrows lifting to meet the high notes (be still, my beating heart). I'll remember his garbled "Are you, Mimi?" to inquire as to my whereabouts, while also asking the question I'd been wondering all along—Are you Mimi?—the answer to which became, over those complicated first years, an emphatic, *Yes, Baby. I am.*

My eyes will flick up to behold that beloved phase of my life, so far behind me as to appear simple, whole, and good, a light without any darkness, just a series of unpolluted joys, and I'll consider it one of life's great injustices that a mother can't stop time. My heart will ache with homesickness, and I'll look back at it all with the dreaminess of a grandparent, musing, *Those were by far my richest days.* And you know what? I will be absolutely right.

ACKNOWLEDGEMENTS

All books are raised by a village, but this is doubly the case for nonfiction since the subject matter required support long before it became art. I am immensely grateful for the villages on either side of this memoir.

Thank you to Phil, my partner in all things, as well as a surprisingly astute editor, even when the names on the page reflect the ones in his life. Thank you to my family for letting me write about them. Although, to be fair, I forgot to ask permission. Thank you to the mom friends whose generous honesty made me feel less alone.

To the person(s) who provided a shipment of formula that gave me the permission, justification, and means to untap my breasts when I'd had enough—thank you.

Thank you to Ioanna Opidee, a brilliant writer and friend, whose early feedback gave me confidence and direction, and to Julia Maggiola, another asset, who encouraged me to shape the voice into one that more closely resembled myself.

Thank you to my agents, Nicki Richesin and Wendy Sherman; my editor at William Morrow, Lucia Macro; and my manager, Katrina Escudero. Their advocacy changed my life.

Thank you to Sarah Zink, whose copyediting saved me from embarrassment.

Thank you to Woodhall Press, for offering a beautiful home for this project, and in particular for the efforts and dedication of Colin, Matt, and Nathaniel.

And of course, thank you to Rowen, my heart and inspiration, whose powerful love made me a mother.

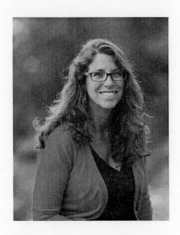

Alena Dillon is the author of *Mercy House*, a Library Journal Best Book of 2020, which has been optioned as a television series produced by Amy Schumer, as well as *The Happiest Girl in the World*, a Good Morning America pick. Her work has appeared in publications including *LitHub*, *River Teeth*, *Slice Magazine*, *The Rumpus*, and *Bustle*. She teaches creative writing and lives on the north shore of Boston with her husband, son, and black lab.

Learn more at AlenaDillon.com